SOUTHERN CALIFORNIA CAMPGROUNDS KEY

D0468748

Other titles in this series:

THE BEST
IN TENT
CAMPING

A GUIDE FOR CAR CAMPERS WHO HATE RVs, CONCRETE SLABS, AND LOUD PORTABLE STEREOS

SOUTHERN CALIFORNIA

FOURTH EDITION

BILL MAI
Revised by Charles Patterson

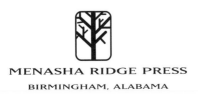

MENASHA RIDGE PRESS
BIRMINGHAM, ALABAMA

For Mary, Casey, John, Kye, and Michael. —Charles Patterson

Library of Congress Cataloging-in-Publication Data

Patterson, Charles.
 The best in tent camping, southern California: a guide for car campers who hate RVs, concrete
slabs, and loud portable stereos/Charles Patterson with Bill Mai. —4th ed.
    p. cm.
 Rev. ed. of: The best in tent camping, southern California/Hans Huber. 3rd ed. c2004.
 ISBN-13: 978-0-89732-675-9
 ISBN-10: 0-89732-675-X
 1. Camping—California, Southern—Guidebooks. 2. Camp sites, facilities, etc.—California,
Southern—Guidebooks. 3. California, Southern—Guidebooks. I. Mai, Bill, 1945— II. Huber, Hans,
1964— Best in tent camping, southern California III. Title.
 GV191.42.C2P38 2008
 917.94'068—dc22
                                    2008037019

Cover and text design by Ian Szymkowiak, Palace Press International, Inc.
Cover photo by Patrick Brady
Cartography by Steve Jones and Charles Patterson
Indexing by Rich Carlson

Menasha Ridge Press
P.O. Box 43673
Birmingham, Alabama 35243
www.menasharidge.com

TABLE OF CONTENTS

THE NORTHERN SIERRAS (continued)

THE SOUTHERN SIERRAS 143

APPENDIXES 000

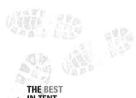

FRIENDS AND FAMILY GET TOGETHER, and pretty soon somebody starts talking about going camping, fishing the streams, and hiking the high country, and suddenly everybody wants to go. Usually the proposed trip fizzles out the next morning because nobody knows quite where to go, or how to arrange it, and nobody wants to end up camping in a little tent on a slab of concrete surrounded by hard-partying RV-ers. Nobody knows a sure good campground, so the whole camping adventure dies on the vine.

Well, that's why you buy this book. You'll discover fifty of the most wonderful spots to tent camp in Southern California and learn how to reserve a spot if necessary, what to expect, and how to get there. All the campgrounds listed here are attractive, clean, safe, and well run.

The best are in the desert, along the coast, and in the mountains. Each of the campgrounds is rated in categories of beauty, site privacy, site spaciousness, quiet, security, and cleanliness, so you pick the best from the best. There's not a loser here. Your choice will depend on what you like and what time of year you want to go camping.

I selected my campgrounds by going camping, by finding the tent-friendly campgrounds, by talking to rangers, and by buttonholing other campers or locals and asking them their favorite spot. I tried to be objective. I reined in my preference for big country pine and boulder-style campgrounds and gave the nod to some campgrounds located deep in the woods. I spaced out the campgrounds, I picked geographically as well as seasonally, and I stayed away from very small campgrounds because even if a few folks show up, they're full.

When you get out and start camping, you'll find your own hit parade of campgrounds. You'll stumble upon all the tiny gems with three or four sites and explore all the fantastic places in the mountains and desert where you can camp anywhere you want. It's a whole new world.

—Bill Mai

THE BEST IN TENT CAMPING

A GUIDE FOR CAR CAMPERS WHO HATE RVs,
CONCRETE SLABS, AND LOUD PORTABLE STEREOS

SOUTHERN CALIFORNIA

FOURTH EDITION

INTRODUCTION

DRIVE FROM A CAMPGROUND BELOW sea level in Death Valley to a campground 10,000 feet up by a glacier in the Sierras in two hours. This diversity is Southern California camping. The Big Sur coast is a wonder of the world. Anza-Borrego State Park is as big as Rhode Island. In the southern mountains, Mt. San Jacinto feels like little Switzerland. Near Julian, you'd swear you were in Vermont. This is a beautiful, beautiful area, and the tent camping is superb. The beaches of the southern coast are legendary.

GEOGRAPHY

For the purposes of this book, Southern California is everything below a line drawn from Santa Cruz across the top of Yosemite National Park to the Nevada border. This area is divided into the Coast, the Desert, the Northern Sierras, and the Southern Sierras.

These four areas represent an amazing diversity in terrain. The Coast includes the 200 miles of sandy beaches north of the Mexican border to above Santa Barbara, and the mountains that parallel the shore above the Los Angeles Basin to Santa Cruz. The Desert, in the southeast corner of California, is a vast and fascinating area of three deserts—Mojave, Colorado, and Sonoran—extending to the Colorado River. The Northern Sierras, or Sierra Nevada, the largest mountain mass in the United States, extends north from the Mojave Desert to Sequoia, Kings Canyon, and Yosemite. The Southern Sierras include the San Bernardinos and other minor ranges that extend southeast into Mexico.

WHERE TO GO AND WHEN

Pleasant camping can be found on the coast year-round. For winter and early spring camping, head for the desert. Between Death Valley National Park, East Mojave National Preserve, Joshua Tree National Park, and Anza-Borrego Desert State Park you could camp all winter and never stay in the same spot twice. Camp the Northern and Southern Sierras in the spring, summer, and fall. The southern beaches are a year-round affair. Never camp the desert in the summer, and camp the mountains in the winter only if you are prepared to go snow camping.

THE RATING SYSTEM

The best campgrounds are rated in various categories—five stars is best, and one star is acceptable. Use the rating system to select the wonderful campground that combines the elements that best suit you.

BEAUTY

While all the campgrounds in this book are beautiful, some are absolutely sensational. They rate five stars, with mountains, streams, waterfalls, and sunsets all conspiring for a drop-dead campground personality. One- to four-star campgrounds are no dogs, either, but possess a less-spectacular beauty that will grow on you.

PRIVACY

Some campgrounds are very well built. The sites are arranged to take maximum advantage of the contour of the land, and the vegetation gives each one the most privacy possible. Good architecture cuts down on the cringe factor when other campers pull in next door. It makes you feel at home from the moment you step out of your car. What a difference!

SPACIOUSNESS

I want flat land to pitch a tent on. I want the flat area far enough from the picnic table so my camping mate can make coffee without waking me and far enough away from the fire pit so the embers don't burn holes in the tent. And I want a view. A view from each campsite is part of the spacious feeling that qualifies a campground for five stars in this category.

QUIET

Quiet is part of beautiful. There's nothing like the sound of a generator or a boom box to ruin an otherwise exquisite campsite. I consider white noise like the roar of a river to improve the quiet rating, since it is natural and it drowns out the sounds of other campers.

SECURITY

Most of the campsites in this guide have campground hosts who keep a good eye on the property, which makes the campground safer than a good neighborhood. The farther the campground is from an urban center, the more secure it is. Of course, you can leave your valuables with the hosts if you're going to be gone for a day or so, but don't leave little things lying around. A blue jay will take off with a pair of sunglasses, and you never can tell what a visiting bear will decide has food value.

CLEANLINESS

Most campgrounds in this guide are well tended. Sometimes, on big weekends, places can get a little rank—not unlike one's kitchen after a big party. I appreciate the little things like the campground host who came around with a rake after each site was vacated to police the place. That particular campground received five stars in the cleanliness department.

GOOD PLANNING

A little planning makes a good camping trip great. First, decide where and when you want to go. Then, phone that district's Ranger Headquarters to make sure the campground is open and that it has water. See if the ranger recommends other campgrounds. See if it's going to be busy. If it is, reserve ahead if possible. All national-forest campgrounds must be reserved at least three to seven days in advance. (*Note:* For all reservable campgrounds in this book, there is a $7.50 fee if you book through **www.reserveamerica.com** or a $9-to-$10 fee if you reserve through **www.recreation.gov.**) Remember, if you arrive and don't like the reserved site, the campground host will move you if another site is available.

Next, get your equipment together. Everybody knows what basics to bring tent camping. A tent (of course), the sleeping bags, a cooler, a stove, pots, utensils, a water jug, matches, a can opener, etc. But, it's those little things that you suddenly wish you had that make a happy camper. The number one objective is a good night's sleep.

Bring earplugs. You need earplugs to get a good snooze. The first night or two out camping, the unfamiliar flap of the tent fabric drives you crazy if you don't have earplugs. Also, a snoring mate sleeping a foot away from you is nighttime hell on earth without earplugs. In addition, earplugs block out all that night nature stuff which interferes with a righteous camper's sleep.

Don't forget to pack your own pillow. A good pillow gets your shoulders off the deck and lets your hips and behind take the weight. Use your clothes bag as an additional pillow (consider inflatable pillows sold at camping stores). Bring a thin foam mattress or buy the self-inflating pads. Buy a spidermat—a device that keeps your pad from slipping on the tent floor and keeps your sleeping bag on top of it. Air mattresses are OK, but susceptible to puncture. Never buy a double air mattress—every time your mate moves you get tossed around. Get a sleeping bag that is good and warm. Nothing is worse than being cold at night, and no sleeping bag is too warm. Bring a sheet so you can sleep under it at first, then crawl into the bag when it gets nippy. Check the weather. If it's going to be cold, remember to bring socks and sweatpants to sleep in. A sweatshirt with a hood is invaluable, since you lose a lot of heat through your head.

Bring a water bottle from which to drink at night. Consequently, a pee jar (a pee pot for ladies) just outside the tent is a great idea. You can stumble outside, use it, and empty it in the toilet in the morning.

Nothing disturbs your Z's like grit inside the tent, so bring something to put outside the tent to clean your feet on. In the woods, a square of AstroTurf works fine. At the seashore or in the desert, a tray full of water in which to dip your feet works best. Bring a small brush for what grit leaks in.

Remember flashlights. The little mini-mags work OK, and if you take off the lens, you can hang them from a tent loop and actually read. Be careful since the little bulb is damn hot and will burn fabric or fingers. But, what works even better is a head lamp. You can buy them at any outdoor store. Just strap the lamp around your head with an adjustable elastic band. Everywhere you look, there's light. They're great for finding stuff, cleaning up in the dark after dinner, and reading. Remember duct tape. "If you can't fix it, duct-tape it" is a camping maxim.

Bring a sponge to clean off the picnic table. A plastic tablecloth is nice, too (bring little pushpins to secure it so it won't blow away). A plastic bowl or a blow-up sink from Basic Designs (around $6 at sports stores) is invaluable for washing dishes. Picnic table benches get mighty hard, so bring a cushion. Buy a cheap lawn chair, and get the inexpensive umbrella that attaches to the back of the chair, so you can sit around the camp out of the sun. While sitting around, you'll want a fly swatter to wreak revenge on a lazy droning fly or two, and mosquito repellent for that irksome gnat in your ear. Bring a little leaf rake to police your camp area. Remember binoculars, a bird book, and a wildflower book, so you can put a name with what you see.

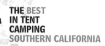

Good water jugs are two-and-a-half-gallon plastic jobs sold in supermarkets. Most have a twist-off cap for refilling. They travel best with their valves up to avoid any leakage. Take a hot shower. Basic Designs (and other outfits) sells a solar shower bag that really works. After a day in the sun sitting on a hot rock, the water is hot! Or, bring along nonscented diaper wipes for a quick sponge bath. They work.

Don't be afraid to ask fellow campers for help or for stuff you might have forgotten. All campers know what it's like to forget basic stuff and love to help fellow campers. There's always a mechanic on vacation camping in next site over when your car won't start or somebody with extra white gas for your stove. Be friendly to your fellow campers. Wave and say "Hi."

The campfire is an important camp event. Stores around the campground sell bundles of wood and, often, the campground host and hostess sell wood. Also, there may be windfalls around the campground from which you can take wood (ask the campground host). You need a good camp saw for that. An absolute essential is a can of charcoal starter fluid. This guarantees a fire even in a driving rain. Naturally, don't forget marshmallows, graham crackers, and chocolate for roasting.

Fix your car up before you go. Nothing can be a bigger bummer than a mechanical breakdown on your way. Have a mechanic check your water hoses and the air pressure in your tires before you load up. Remember, your car will be loaded down with stuff, and this will put a strain on your tires and cooling system. Bring an extra fan belt. Nothing can shut down the car like a snapped fan belt that you have to special-order from Japan. Even if you don't know a fan belt from third base, bring one. Somebody will come along who knows how to install it. Make sure your spare tire is correctly inflated. Mishap #999 is when you put on your spare, let the car down, and find out the spare is flat.

If you fish, be sure to get a license and display it. Fishing without a license is a misdemeanor, punishable by a maximum fine of $1,000 and/or six months in jail. On your way into the campground, stop at a local store and find out what the folks are using for bait. Buy it. This will save you a lot of experimentation and probably provide you with a good meal.

Remember the bears! We have few mosquitoes here in Southern California, but a lot of black bears. Never leave your cooler out. Put it in the trunk or disguise it with a blanket if you have a hatchback or a van. Don't eat in your tent. Take all cosmetics, soap, etc. and put them in the car. Disguise them, too. A bear will rip off a car door to get a tube of lip balm. Bring a small bottle of bleach to wipe down your picnic table at night—bears don't like bleach (but, don't put too much faith in this!). If a bear raids your camp looking for food, shoo him away like you would a naughty dog. Don't worry. Even the boldest bears don't go into tents unless they smell food.

Think about dispersed camping. With a fire permit, a shovel, and a bucket of water, you can camp just about anywhere in the national forests (consult Ranger District Headquarters) and in Anza-Borrego Desert State Park.

The fire permit costs nothing, and there are miles and miles of fire roads and lumber roads you can explore to find the dispersed campground of your dreams.

SETTLING IN

When you come into a campground, be aware of a certain psychological barrier. This is a new place. Suddenly, you've driven all this way, and the campground doesn't look that hot. You feel disappointed. You feel like the "new kid at school." The other campers look up from their game of gin rummy and hope you won't camp next to them as you drive around the campground loops and look helplessly at the open sites. Nothing looks good enough.

Park your car. Pull into the first available site that could possibly do. Then, walk around the campground. You have half an hour to decide before you pick your site and pay. Once you get out and walk, you'll break through that "new kid at school" dilemma and soon feel like you're a part of the place. It's odd. Suddenly, you don't mind camping next to the gin rummy players. You realize that this is your campground as well as theirs. By the next morning, the whole place will feel like home, and the gin rummy players will seem like the best of neighbors. You won't understand why you didn't immediately recognize this campground as the best.

When you plan a camping trip, try to stay in one campground for at least three days. Stay one day, and you end up spending most of your time packing and unpacking and getting familiar with the campground. Stay three days, and you'll relax and have fun.

Go tent camping. Live in paradise for a few days. Camping makes you want to sin like the damned, sleep like the righteous, and hike like the last of the great American walkers. It's a balm for the weary soul!

BEST OF SOUTHERN CALIFORNIA CAMPGROUNDS

BEST FOR PRIVACY
1 ARROYO SALADO PRIMITIVE CAMPGROUND
2 LA JOLLA VALLEY HIKE-IN CAMPGROUND
3 LITTLE BLAIR VALLEY PRIMITIVE CAMPGROUND
4 TRAPPER SPRINGS CAMPGROUND
5 VERMILION CAMPGROUND

BEST FOR SPACIOUSNESS
1 MARION MOUNTAIN CAMPGROUND
2 TRAPPER SPRINGS CAMPGROUND
3 FOUR JEFFREY AND SABRINA CAMPGROUNDS
4 COLD SPRINGS CAMPGROUND
5 ARROYO SALADO PRIMITIVE CAMPGROUND

BEST FOR QUIET
1 DARK CANYON CAMPGROUND
2 LA JOLLA VALLEY HIKE-IN CAMPGROUND
3 MID HILLS CAMPGROUND
4 COLD SPRINGS CAMPGROUND
5 WHITE WOLF CAMPGROUND

BEST FOR SECURITY
1 LAGUNA CAMPGROUND
2 TRAPPER SPRINGS CAMPGROUND
3 MINARET FALLS CAMPGROUND
4 SADDLEBAG BUTTE STATE PARK CAMPGROUND
5 MESQUITE SPRINGS CAMPGROUND

BEST FOR BEAUTY
1 ANDREW MOLERA STATE PARK CAMPGROUND
2 MONTAÑA DE ORO SATE PARK CAMPGROUND
3 WHITE TANK CAMPGROUND
4 ATWELL MILL CAMPGROUND
5 HORSE MEADOW CAMPGROUND

BEST FOR CLEANLINESS
1 LOWER PEPPERMINT CAMPGROUND
2 MORAINE CAMPGROUND
3 TWIN LAKES CAMPGROUND
4 HANNA FLAT CAMPGROUND
5 PINNACLES CAMPGROUND

BEST FOR WHEELCHAIRS
1 LOWER PEPPERMINT CAMPGROUND
2 MORAINE CAMPGROUND
3 TWIN LAKES CAMPGROUND
4 HANNA FLAT CAMPGROUND
5 PINNACLES CAMPGROUND

BEST FOR FISHING
1 SADDLEBAG LAKE CAMPGROUND
2 TWIN LAKES CAMPGROUND
3 BUCKEYE CAMPGROUND
4 VERMILION CAMPGROUND
5 THORNHILL BROOME BEACH CAMPGROUND

BEST FOR HIKING
1 WHITE WOLF CAMPGROUND
2 BIG SYCAMORE CANYON CAMPGROUND
3 MALIBU CREEK STATE PARK CAMPGROUND
4 SADDLEBAG LAKE CAMPGROUND
5 TRUMBULL LAKE CAMPGROUND

BEST FOR PADDLING
1 VERMILLION CAMPGROUND
2 LEO CARRILLO STATE BEACH CAMPGROUND
3 TWIN LAKES CAMPGROUND
4 RANCHERIA CAMPGROUND
5 TILLIE CREEK CAMPGROUND

BEST FOR SWIMMING
1 LEO CARRILLO STATE BEACH CAMPGROUND
2 BUCKEYE CAMPGROUND
3 HORSE MEADOW CAMPGROUND
4 McGRATH STATE BEACH CAMPGROUND
5 EL CAPITAN STATE PARK CAMPGROUND

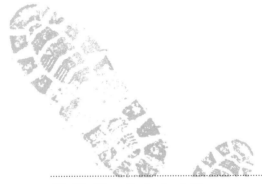

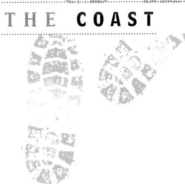

THE **COAST**

01
ANDREW MOLERA
STATE PARK
CAMPGROUND

GO TO **ANDREW MOLERA STATE PARK** and walk the 1-mile trail to the ocean. The beach is awesome—4 miles of Big Sur's longest sandy stretches. Find sea fig, sand verbena, silverwood, and beach primrose on the side of the dunes. On the bluffs, look for seaside painted cups, sea lettuce, beach sagewort, and coast eriogonum. On my last trip to Andrew Molera, I brought a plant-identification book and actually identified a few of the species named above.

I had even better luck with the birds. I saw black long-necked cormorants off Molera Point, willits, and a great blue heron. Look for the mass of tiny sanderlings that flow in behind the waves to feed before the breakers come again. They are looking for small sand crabs.

When I visited Andrew Molera in March, I hiked out on the Headlands Trail and saw a pod of gray whales heading south. Also, keep an eye out for otters. They are members of the weasel family, with slim bodies, high hips, broad heads, and short furry tails. Weighing about 80 pounds, the otter has feet that function like hands, so they can use rocks as hammers to smash shells. They have lovely, light whiskers and live together, in groups called rafts, in the kelp beds a mile or so from shore. This is where the mothers teach their babies to swim down and get food from the ocean floor below. They also teach them to hide among the bulbs of the bull kelp, so the great white shark can't find them and eat them.

Once thought extinct, the otters are still an endangered species. The last count was around 2,000 otters (including pups) living along the California coast—ranging from Vandenberg Air Force Base in Santa Barbara County to the San Francisco Bay.

Storms that separate pups from their mothers are a big problem, since pups can't survive alone. The

> *Andrew Molera has it all—Big Sur, a river, the sea, mountains, and tent camping in a grassy meadow.*

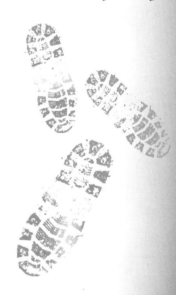

RATINGS

Beauty: ✩ ✩ ✩ ✩ ✩
Privacy: ✩ ✩ ✩ ✩
Spaciousness: ✩ ✩ ✩ ✩
Quiet: ✩ ✩ ✩ ✩
Security: ✩ ✩ ✩ ✩
Cleanliness: ✩ ✩ ✩ ✩

ADDRESS:	Andrew Molera State Park Campground c/o Big Sur Station #1 Big Sur, CA 93920
OPERATED BY:	California State Parks
INFORMATION:	(831) 667-2315; www.parks.ca.gov
OPEN:	Year-round
SITES:	24
EACH SITE HAS:	Limited picnic tables, fireplaces
ASSIGNMENT:	First come, first served; no reservations
REGISTRATION:	Self-registration at campground
FACILITIES:	Water, flush toilets, firewood for sale
PARKING:	In parking lot; walk to campground; $2–$4 developed; $4–$14 undeveloped
FEE:	$10
ELEVATION:	Near sea level
RESTRICTIONS:	*Pets:* Not allowed *Fires:* In fireplaces *Alcohol:* No restrictions *Vehicles:* Not allowed in campgrounds *Other:* 3-day stay limit (must vacate for 7 days to return)

lucky ones are washed ashore and found by nice folks, who take them to the Monterey Bay Aquarium for rehabilitation. Here, they are paired with a surrogate mother and are taught to swim, hunt food, and groom their fur. The surrogates are not other otters, but scientists in diving gear.

From the bluffs, the ocean reflects incredible colors. The purer the water, the deeper the color—this prismatic show all depends on how the sunlight is scattered by the water molecules. The old lava beds of Point Sur show the rainbow shades, and the kelp beds turn spots of blue to deep green. The light blue and turquoise along the cliffs are caused by the surf forcing air into the water. Plumes of red, brown, and green are the streams pouring Santa Lucia silt into the ocean.

The camping in Andrew Molera is pure tent camping. The sites are in a beautiful, grassy meadow a short walk from the parking lot (the last time I was there I had a cooler heavy with ice, beer, and soda, and I wished I'd brought one of those airport dollies you use to carry heavy suitcases). There are flush toilets and piped-water spigots set around the meadow. There are 24 campsites. The crowd was young and very friendly. And the price ($10) is right as rain. There is a three-day limit, and then you have to stay away for seven days before returning.

The Big Sur River meanders through Andrew Molera, offering sandy banks for sunbathing and shallow water for wading. But the ocean here is rough, cold, and often windy. Only the makeshift huts built by sunbathers let you brave the afternoon wind. Beware of rogue waves, and don't get blocked by the tides.

There is no excuse for not having a campfire at Andrew Molera. You are permitted to collect up to 50 pounds of driftwood from the beach. All other wood in the park is protected. Really lazy people can purchase firewood at the stores along CA 1, or you can even purchase it at the campground.

You'll find good hiking east of the highway. As you climb the East Molera Trail, see madrone, coast live oak, canyon oak, and then redwood at the crest of the ridge. Look for Indian paintbrush, red elderberry,

MAP

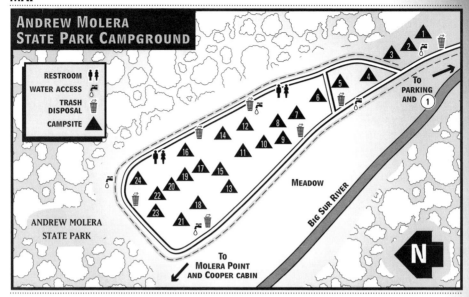

ANDREW MOLERA STATE PARK CAMPGROUND

RESTROOM
WATER ACCESS
TRASH DISPOSAL
CAMPSITE

To PARKING AND (1)

MEADOW

BIG SUR RIVER

ANDREW MOLERA STATE PARK

To MOLERA POINT AND COOPER CABIN

N

and red maids. Keep going when the trail ends and reach the South Fork Little Sur River down the other side of the ridge.

GETTING THERE

From San Francisco, drive south on CA 1 to Carmel, then drive 21 miles south on CA 1 to Andrew Molera State Park on the right.

GPS COORDINATES

UTM Zone (WGS84) 10S
Easting 602174
Northing 4015793
Latitude N 36° 16' 54"
Longtitude W 106° 51 '44"

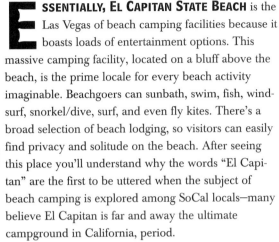

> *Many SoCal locals
> believe El Capitan is
> far and away the
> ultimate campground
> in California.*

ESSENTIALLY, EL CAPITAN STATE BEACH is the Las Vegas of beach camping facilities because it boasts loads of entertainment options. This massive camping facility, located on a bluff above the beach, is the prime locale for every beach activity imaginable. Beachgoers can sunbath, swim, fish, windsurf, snorkel/dive, surf, and even fly kites. There's a broad selection of beach lodging, so visitors can easily find privacy and solitude on the beach. After seeing this place you'll understand why the words "El Capitan" are the first to be uttered when the subject of beach camping is explored among SoCal locals—many believe El Capitan is far and away the ultimate campground in California, period.

The attraction of El Capitan has everything to do with its geography. The campsites are perched in a grove of oak trees atop a bluff above the shoreline. Most sites have unobstructed ocean views, and many offer natural privacy. Although there are no sites on the sandy beach, several easy-to-find trails lead down to various sections of shoreline. El Capitan State Beach lies on a point, and surfers will love the point break to the east of the sites when the swells are up. During low tides, tide pools will appear around the east end of the point for beach walkers to explore.

There are always a few among us who don't particularly enjoy the ocean—but they needn't stay home, because there's a great bike path that runs for 2 miles, connecting El Capitan State Beach with Refugio State Beach. The path allows beachgoers easy access to the entire length of shoreline between the two parks. As a matter of fact, you'll be stunned to see so many kids on bikes at El Capitan. Please be wary of them when driving through the park. Ocean-haters and hikers alike can explore the hiking trails of the

RATINGS

Beauty: ✪ ✪ ✪ ✪ ✪
Privacy: ✪ ✪ ✪
Spaciousness: ✪ ✪ ✪ ✪
Quiet: ✪ ✪ ✪
Security: ✪ ✪ ✪
Cleanliness: ✪ ✪ ✪ ✪

nearby El Capitan Canyon, located to the north, on the other side of US 101.

The ample shade among the campsites makes the beach camping manageable for people sensitive to the sun. Those who've spent a whole day under the sun understand this—it's very easy to become overwhelmed with sun-spawned beach fatigue and literally get "beached out." El Capitan allows visitors to fully escape the beach environment in the oak groves. Inside several sites it's quite possible to forget the beach entirely, because the immediate surroundings look like the typical chaparral environment of the interior.

Anyone who's spent time on the waters off Southern California knows that one of mankind's most ferocious predators lurks beneath—the great white shark. Frankly speaking, the waters off southern California are great-white habitat. Attacks, however, are extremely rare. Great whites are feared more for their intimidating appearance than their actual deadliness. Bull and tiger sharks have attacked and killed far more people worldwide than great whites, but they get none of the credit because they don't look as menacing and weren't in the film and book *Jaws*. The total number of great-white-shark fatalities in California history is difficult to calculate, and estimates differ, but it's safe to assume that just more than 100 people have died from great-white attacks in California since 1900. This number pales in comparison to the hundreds of thousands of people in the water every year. To say there's nothing to fear would be a lie, but consider this: more people are killed each year by falling coconuts than sharks worldwide. Yet, nobody's afraid of visiting tropical locales where coconut trees are common, but many won't get in the water because of sharks. Kind of silly, isn't it?

Perhaps the icing on the cake for El Capitan is the fact that the highway (US 101) is far enough from the grounds to be drowned out of audible existence by the lapping surf below, unlike any other beach camping facilities in SoCal. El Capitan truly is the "captain" of SoCal's state beaches, and it's baffling this place isn't dotted with opulent beach houses instead of being open to the public. All this ecstasy comes at a price— the usual six-month waiting period for reservations.

KEY INFORMATION

ADDRESS: El Capitan State Beach
10 Refugio Beach Road
Goleta, CA 93117

OPERATED BY: California State Parks

INFORMATION: (805) 968-1033; www.parks.ca.gov

OPEN: Year-round

SITES: 132

EACH SITE: Picnic table, fire ring

ASSIGNMENT: Reservations can be made online via www.reserveamerica.com, or by calling (800) 444-7275.

REGISTRATION: Self-registration if park entrance station is closed

FACILITIES: Bathrooms, running water, showers

PARKING: On site

FEE: $25; $20 off-season (Dec. 1–Feb. 28); $7.50 reservation fee

ELEVATION: Sea level

RESTRICTIONS: *Pets:* Dogs must be kept on a 6-foot leash at all times, are not permitted on the beach or in buildings, and must be inside vehicle or tent at night.
Fires: Permitted within established fire rings
Alcohol: No restrictions

MAP

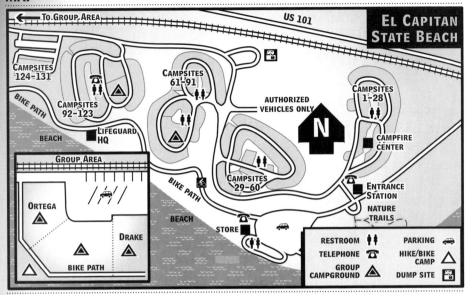

GETTING THERE

El Capitan State Beach is hard to miss—it's located 17 miles northwest of Santa Barbara off US 101, clearly marked with large signs.

GPS COORDINATES

UTM Zone (WGS 84) 11S

Easting 773367

Northing 3817214

Latitude N 34° 27' 37"

Longitude W 120° 01' 26"

03
FREMONT PEAK STATE PARK CAMPGROUND

FREMONT **P**EAK **S**TATE **P**ARK is deliriously pretty in April and May, when the spring grasses are green and feathery and the flowers are blooming. It's a great place to go when the coast is socked in with fog. Climb to the peak and look out over both the richest farmland and the richest marine area in the world.

The drive up to the park from San Juan Bautista is alternately lovely, chilling, and lovely again. At first, you take a winding, old country road out of the valley and up into oaks draped with mistletoe. Then you burst into Road Warrior country. On the left is the Hollister Hills State Vehicular Recreation Area, where off-road enthusiasts bring their vehicles. It's a land of tire-ripped hills and torched brush. Scary. But persevere and you arrive at the mountaintop to enter Fremont Peak State Park with its oaks, pines, and incredible views.

The camping here is primitive and best suited for tents. All the sites are roomy, grassy, and shaded by oaks. There is potable water, and each site boasts an incredible view of Monterey Bay. However, it is best to avoid the area in the summer, when Gavilan Peak is overrun by nasty little biting flies.

Fremont Peak State Park is actually not situated on Fremont Peak, but on Gavilan Peak. The expansive view from Gavilan prompted John C. Fremont to build a fort there one fateful day in 1846. California, then a territory of Mexico, was seething. The Mexican government wanted to get rid of the American settlers, who were forming ragtag armies to take over the territory. In additon, Native Americans were arming and trying to retake their former lands. Into the middle of this rode John C. Fremont, a captain of the Topographical Engineers of the United States, to map the California Trail.

Come to Fremont Peak State Park for spring camping and to San Juan Bautista for California's yesterdays.

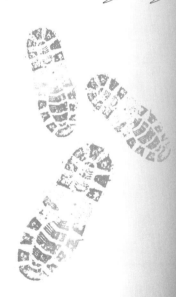

RATINGS

Beauty: ☆ ☆ ☆ ☆ ☆
Privacy: ☆ ☆ ☆
Spaciousness: ☆ ☆ ☆ ☆
Quiet: ☆ ☆ ☆ ☆
Security: ☆ ☆ ☆
Cleanliness: ☆ ☆ ☆

KEY INFORMATION

ADDRESS:	Fremont Peak State Park Campground P.O. Box 787 San Juan Bautista, CA 95045
OPERATED BY:	California State Parks
INFORMATION:	(831) 623-42551; www.parks.ca.gov; at the San Juan Bautista State Historic Park
OPEN:	March 1–November 30
SITES:	25
EACH SITE HAS:	Picnic table, fire ring
ASSIGNMENT:	Online at www.reserveamerica.com or (800) 444-7275
REGISTRATION:	At entrance
FACILITIES:	Water, pit toilets, wheelchair-accessible sites
PARKING:	At site
FEE:	$15; $11 off-season, plus $7.50 reservation fee
ELEVATION:	2,750 feet
RESTRICTIONS:	*Pets:* Dogs on leash only in campground; not allowed on trails *Fires:* In fire rings (no firewood available at campgrounds) *Alcohol:* No restrictions *Vehicles:* 18-foot trailers, 26-foot RVs *Other:* $1 day-use fee; keep food stored in vehicle when not in campsite to prevent feral pig depredation

Jose Castro, the Mexican governor, ordered Fremont and his group of Delaware Native Americans and hard-bitten frontiersmen to leave the territory. Fremont refused. Cheekily, he marched his men up Gavilan Peak and built a rough log fort within plain sight of General Castro's headquarters in San Juan Bautista. When Fremont raised the American flag up a stripped sapling, his men cheered, but General Castro was livid. He posted a proclamation:

Fellow Citizens: A band of robbers commanded by a captain of the United States Army, J. C. Fremont, have without respect to the laws and authorities of the department daringly introduced themselves into the country and disobeyed the orders both of your commander-in-chief and of the prefect of the district.

Castro summoned a band of Mexican cavalrymen from Monterey north to San Juan.

Fremont set an ambush for the cavalrymen, but at the last minute, the Mexican officers inexplicably ordered their troops back to Monterey. Meanwhile, on the peak, the westerly wind kicked up and blew the crude flagpole down. Taking this as a sign, Fremont abandoned his fort and grudgingly retreated.

General Castro called the Americans "cowards and poor guests," and the incident was over, but both Fremont and Castro would play giant roles in the subsequent turnover of Mexican California to the United States.

Near the campground is the Fremont Park Observatory, with a 30-inch reflecting telescope. They have special programs in the spring and fall. Write the Fremont Park Observatory Association, P.O. Box 787, San Juan Bautista, CA 95045, or phone (831) 623-2465 for a schedule.

A good hike to the peak begins in the parking lot. You'll see a road and a trail. The trail, signed with a hiker's symbol, leads to the observatory. Take the road for a short distance, then join the signed Peak Trail, which circles the mountain.

On the high ridges, see Coulter pine and madrone. The northern slopes are full of manzanita, toyon, and scrub oak, and the southern slopes spill

MAP

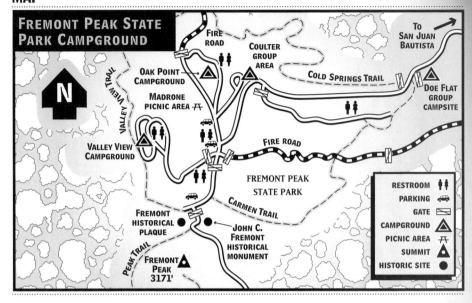

FREMONT PEAK STATE PARK CAMPGROUND

FIRE ROAD

COULTER GROUP AREA

To SAN JUAN BAUTISTA

OAK POINT CAMPGROUND

COLD SPRINGS TRAIL

DOE FLAT GROUP CAMPSITE

MADRONE PICNIC AREA

VALLEY VIEW TRAIL

FIRE ROAD

VALLEY VIEW CAMPGROUND

FREMONT PEAK STATE PARK

CARMEN TRAIL

FREMONT HISTORICAL PLAQUE

JOHN C. FREMONT HISTORICAL MONUMENT

PEAK TRAIL

FREMONT PEAK 3171'

RESTROOM	
PARKING	
GATE	
CAMPGROUND	
PICNIC AREA	
SUMMIT	
HISTORIC SITE	

over with grasses and wildflowers. Don't forget your binoculars.

Visit San Juan Bautista, once the district headquarters of the northern half of Alta, California. The 1906 earthquake destroyed half the town, and soon cows grazed on the Plaza. As Will Durant once said, "Civilization exists by geological consent, subject to change without notice." San Juan slept until it was resurrected by benefactors of the old mission and the California Department of Parks and Recreation. I can't count the number of times I have driven US 101 and passed by San Juan Bautista. However, after one visit, I'm a believer. The Old Mission and the Plaza have been lovingly restored.

GETTING THERE

From L.A., drive 330 miles north on US 101 to Salinas, then continue north on US 101 a few miles and turn east on CA 156. Turn right (south) on Juan Canyon Road and drive 11 miles to the campground along a narrow, winding road.

GPS COORDINATES

UTM Zone (WGS 84) 10S
Easting 635567
Northing 3983895
Latitude N 35° 59' 24"
Longtitude W 121° 29' 46"

KIRK CREEK AND PLASKETT CREEK CAMPGROUNDS

> *Come for the huge cliffs of jade. Stay for great camping and hiking in the mountains.*

KIRK CREEK AND PLASKETT CREEK campgrounds are like fraternal twins. They occupy the most isolated stretch of CA 1, north of San Simeon and south of Big Sur. About 5 miles apart, on the best stretch of Los Padres National Forest coastline, these campgrounds offer the most relaxed camping on the entire Southern California coast.

Kirk Creek lies on a bluff overlooking the ocean. Set in gorse—a spiny, yellow-flowered bush—it gets quite a lot of wind. Of course, the view is shockingly immediate—as if you are suspended over the ocean itself. The sites are separated and private until you stand up; the brush surrounding the sites is about chest high. This does, however, give you some relief from the oceanic blasts. Thankfully, there's a fence along the edge of the precipice. Just south, there are goat trails leading down to a rocky point and a sandy cove at low tide. Navigate these trails during the daylight hours.

Plaskett Creek Campground is oriented more toward small RVs, with larger and more level sites. Plaskett is farther from the beach, behind a line of Monterey pines, and not as subject to the ocean's gusty blasts. The area is nice and grassy. The sites are roomier, but not as private without the impenetrable gorse cover of Kirk.

I love both campgrounds. Many CA 1 tourists speed through this area, because you feel as if you're between the devil and the deep blue sea here.

The nearby U.S. Forest Service station at Pacific Valley is primarily used as a fire station. An area map and other information are posted outside the station. The station does not have regularly scheduled hours of operation, but when personnel are on duty they are available to assist visitors. Maps are for sale.

There is mountain hiking in the mountains

RATINGS

Beauty: ✿ ✿ ✿ ✿ ✿
Privacy: ✿ ✿ ✿ ✿ ✿
Spaciousness: ✿ ✿ ✿ ✿ ✿
Quiet: ✿ ✿ ✿ ✿ ✿
Security: ✿ ✿ ✿
Cleanliness: ✿ ✿ ✿ ✿ ✿

directly east of the campground. Though the hiking is good and the weather is cool, the big draw here is the beach. Go to aptly named Jade Cove to see the huge cliffs made entirely of jade. What a magical experience! Walk down from the picnic area, over the cattle gate to the beach, and, as the stairs hit the sand, you'll see the jade on the left. Then, continue south on the beach. I came here once as a child and was overwhelmed by the magic of the green rock, the huge whips of kelp, the surf and white spume, and the shockingly cold water.

Child or adult, no one can help but react viscerally to the primordial beauty of this coastline. We are all drawn to the sea. Why? Our bodies are mostly water, and our blood has the same saline content as the sea. We are carried in water in the womb. Another explanation reaches further back than that, to a dark age of humanity, known as the Pliocene Gap, from 4 million to 7 million years ago. Herbivorous apes went into it, and carnivorous ape-men came out of it. There are no fossils to explain the transformation, but one au courant theory holds that our ancestors passed through a water-living stage.

This would explain the layer of subcutaneous fat unique to humans, as well as the partial webbing between our fingers and toes. Our spines are more flexible than apes', allowing us to swim, and we have a sense of balance equal to sea lions. We are streamlined (having very little hair) and can hold our breath for as long as three and a half minutes. Humans, like other marine animals, also possess a diving reflex that closes down our airways and slows our heart to half speed. Human babies, unlike apes, automatically hold their breath under water. Theorists believe that the sea-ape got a taste for fish and shellfish and returned to land with an expanded taste for meat.

For another ocean experience, go pebble-hunting on the San Simeon coast. Find jadite and brown-and-green chert pebbles. Native Americans fashioned arrowheads from chert. The best hunting is on Moonstone Beach. Turn off CA 1 in Cambria at Windsor Boulevard, then go northwest about 0.4 miles on Moonstone Beach Drive to the state beach parking

ADDRESS:	Kirk Creek and Plaskett Creek Campgrounds Los Padres National Forest 6755 Hollister Avenue, Suite 150 Goleta, CA 93117
OPERATED BY:	U.S. Forest Service
INFORMATION:	(805) 968-6640; www.fs.fed.us/r5/lospadres
OPEN:	Year-round
SITES:	Kirk 33, Plaskett 45
EACH SITE HAS:	Picnic table, fireplace
ASSIGNMENT:	First come, first served; no reservations in Kirk Creek
REGISTRATION:	At entrance, or reserve by phone (Plaskett) at (877) 444-6777 or online at www.recreation.gov.
FACILITIES:	Water, flush toilets
PARKING:	At site
FEE:	$22 plus $9 reservation fee
ELEVATION:	Near sea level
RESTRICTIONS:	*Pets:* On leash only *Fires:* In fireplaces *Alcohol:* No restrictions *Vehicles:* Small RVs *Others:* 14-day stay limit

MAP

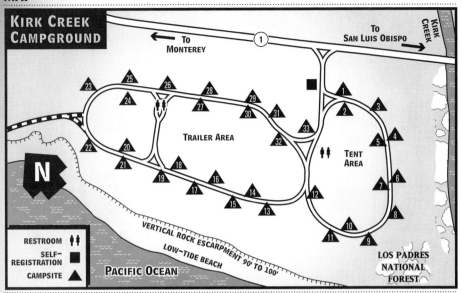

KIRK CREEK CAMPGROUND

To MONTEREY ←

① To SAN LUIS OBISPO →

KIRK CREEK

23 25 26 28 29 24 27 30 31

TRAILER AREA

1 3 2 33 5 4

TENT AREA

22 20 18 21 19 16 17 14 12 6 7 8 15 13 10 9 11

N

RESTROOM 👫
SELF-REGISTRATION ■
CAMPSITE ▲

VERTICAL ROCK ESCARPMENT 90' TO 100'
LOW-TIDE BEACH

PACIFIC OCEAN

LOS PADRES NATIONAL FOREST

GETTING THERE

From San Francisco, drive south on CA 1 through Monterey to Lucia. Then drive 4 miles farther south on CA 1 to Kirk Creek Campground on the right. Plaskett Creek Campground is 5.5 miles still farther south from Kirk Creek Campground. After you pass the Ranger Station, Plaskett Creek will be on your left.

area. Go down to the beach and walk northwest to the cliff. Also, try the beach at Pico Creek, 2.5 miles north of San Simeon Beach Campground.

In July and August, be sure to get to Kirk or Plaskett by Thursday. They fill up, and no reservations are accepted for groups of fewer than 25. Tent campers should stop at the Ranger Station between the two campgrounds and get directions to dispersed camping areas in the nearby wilderness.

MAP

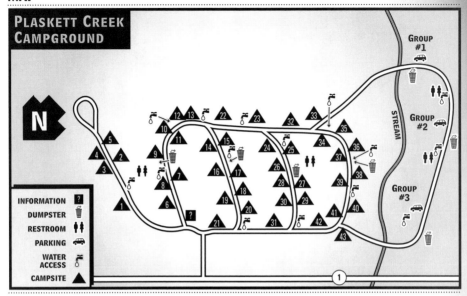

GPS COORDINATES

UTM Zone (WGS 84)	10S
Easting	635567
Northing	3983895
Latitude	N 35° 59' 24"
Longtitude	W 121° 29 ' 46"

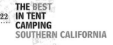

05
LEO CARRILLO STATE BEACH CAMPGROUND

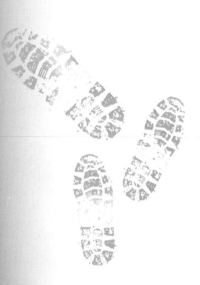

> *After one visit to Leo Carrillo, you'll be hooked.*

AT FIRST GLANCE, the Leo Carrillo State Beach campgrounds look very similar to the nearby facility at Big Sycamore Canyon, but Leo Carrillo caters to a different clientele. While it lacks the world-class mountain-bike trails of Sycamore, Leo Carrillo State Beach may be the ultimate destination for lovers of everything aquatic—surfing, windsurfing, kite-surfing, scuba diving, sportfishing, kayaking, etc. Leo Carrillo is prime ground for all these pursuits, and even more.

Unlike Sycamore's main beach, Leo Carrillo's is protected by rocky obstructions that block the open ocean surge and provide safer waters for casual swimmers at the main beach. It's also a sunbather's paradise, with almost 2 miles of sparsely inhabited sandy beach to the south providing plenty of space for privacy and summertime bliss. The beach is highly picturesque and even offers an easily accessible sea cave. At low tide, amazing assortments of tide pools are exposed, giving the kids plenty to do.

Just as they do at Sycamore Canyon, campers access the beaches by walking through a creek-wash tunnel underneath the Pacific Coast Highway. Across the highway, 140 tent campsites are arrayed along the narrows of Arroyo Sequit Creek. The sites are spacious, and many offer natural borders and privacy with adequate separation between sites, along with plenty of shade provided by tall sycamore trees.

The area surrounding the campsites is a peaceful riparian landscape, much like Malibu's Surfrider Beach and Topanga Beach would have looked before urban development. Giving your skin a break with an afternoon nap under the shade of the sycamores is a highly effective destressor. There are also great hiking trails to explore, though mountain biking on many of these trails is prohibited.

RATINGS

Beauty: ✩ ✩ ✩ ✩ ✩
Privacy: ✩ ✩ ✩
Spaciousness: ✩ ✩ ✩ ✩
Quiet: ✩ ✩ ✩
Security: ✩ ✩ ✩
Cleanliness: ✩ ✩ ✩ ✩ ✩

Leo Carrillo State Beach was named after Hollywood character actor Leo Carrillo (August 6, 1880–September 10, 1961), who played typecast roles most of his career, but was most remembered for his role as Pancho in the 1950s TV show *The Cisco Kid.* The beach wasn't, however, given his name to honor his contributions to entertainment: Carrillo was also an influential conservationist and preservationist. While serving on the California Beach and Parks commission, Carrillo helped add Hearst Castle in San Simeon and Anza-Borrego Desert to California's state-park inventory. His efforts are honored elsewhere in California— Leo Carrillo Elementary School in Westminster and Leo Carrillo Ranch Historic Park in Carlsbad. The Hollywood connection doesn't end with Carrillo; the beach named after him has been a popular locale for high-profile film and photographic shoots for many years, the most memorable being *Grease, The Karate Kid,* and *Point Break.*

Those unfamiliar with California coastal waters may find themselves startled by the chilliness of the water, even during the hottest months of the year. At its warmest, the waters off Leo Carrillo State Beach seldom exceed 65°F and drop to the mid-50s or lower during the winter and spring. Oceanic currents are to blame for this—the California Current is essentially a massive river of cold water that moves south along the Pacific Coast. The water is cold because it originates in the freezing Pacific Northwest. Contrarily, the coastal waters of the eastern United States are significantly warmer during the summer, because the Gulf Stream, originating in the balmy Gulf of Mexico—moves north, carrying warm waters up the East Coast year-round. Amphibious folks will find themselves in wet suits frequently. Full-body suits are suitable for winter surfing; a 3-millimeter thickness will suffice. Skin divers will do OK with the same gear but will probably also need neoprene hoods to stay warm. Scuba diving requires 7-millimeter suits, gloves, hoods, and booties at all times.

Camping at Leo Carrillo offers greatness in two environments—the beach and the wilderness. Understandably, there's a six-month waiting list for reservations during the peak season (March 1 to November

ADDRESS:	35000 West Pacific Coast Highway Malibu, CA 90265
OPERATED BY:	California State Parks
INFORMATION:	(818) 880-0363; www.parks.ca.gov
OPEN:	Year-round
SITES:	135
EACH SITE:	Picnic tables, fire ring
ASSIGNMENT:	Reservations can be made online via www.reserve america.com, or by calling (800) 444-7275.
REGISTRATION:	Self-registration if park entrance station is closed
FACILITIES:	Running water, bathrooms, showers, camp store
PARKING:	$10
FEE:	$25 peak season, $20 off-season, $7.50 reservation fee
ELEVATION:	Sea level
RESTRICTIONS:	*Pets:* Dogs must be kept on a 6-foot leash at all times, are not permitted on beach or in buildings, and must be inside vehicle or tent at night.

MAP

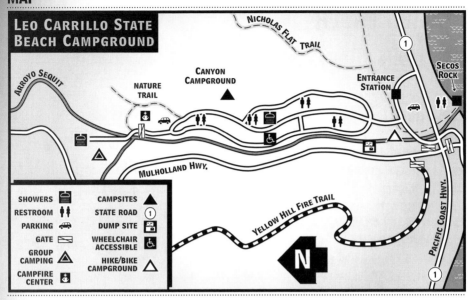

GETTING THERE

Leo Carrillo State Beach is highly visible from the Pacific Coast Highway. From Santa Monica, head northwest on the Pacific Coast Highway approximately 26.5 miles, after which Leo Carrillo State Beach will appear on the right side of the road, clearly marked with signs. From Oxnard, look for Leo Carrillo State Beach after 16 miles on the Pacific Coast Highway heading southeast.

30). Book your site now so you can rediscover SoCal beach splendor. After one visit, you'll be addicted, camping at Leo Carrillo every year even if you're a local and thought you were jaded and somehow bored with SoCal's beaches. If a campsite can't be secured until the following summer, a day trip to this cherished locale is highly recommended and worth every penny spent on gasoline.

GPS COORDINATES

UTM Zone (WGS 84) 11S

Easting 321511

Northing 3769161

Latitude N 34° 05' 53"

Longitude W 118° 56' 01"

06
MALIBU CREEK STATE PARK CAMPGROUND

S **ITUATED ON A BIG HUNK** of the most coveted real estate in Southern California and surrounded by the rapidly encroaching megalopolis of the L.A. area, Malibu Creek State Park Campground is a precious gem. It is spectacular! With sections once owned by Bob Hope, Ronald Reagan, and 20th Century Fox, the park now covers more than 7,000 acres. This is a great place to tent camp in fall, winter, and spring. Protected by a mountain range from the springtime fog blahs that hit the beaches in Southern California, Malibu Creek State Park is situated between two major tourist thoroughfares—CA 1 and US 101. It's just 40 miles down the hill to Malibu and all the wonderful beaches. You're also near Santa Barbara on US 101 and Universal City to the east.

You'll find safe mountain biking and hiking, so this is a great place to bring children camping. It's also a good first night's camp if you are flying into LAX, and a good escape from L.A. if you happen to live there. I've camped at Malibu Creek State Park several times over Saturday night with my wife, eaten at the nearby Saddle Peak Lodge (excellent food), then ducked back to our humble tent for a weekend combining the high life and the great outdoors.

High season at the campground begins with spring break and goes through the end of September. Since Malibu Creek can get crowded, be sure to come early on weekends during the summer. The ranger recommended arriving by noon on Friday to reserve a spot for a summer weekend. The campground is very clean, well patrolled, and well maintained, but the sites themselves are unremarkable. The incredible vista and the "neighborhood" are what make this a fun camping experience.

> *A good base camp from which to explore Los Angeles; with easy hiking and bicycling, it's also good for kids.*

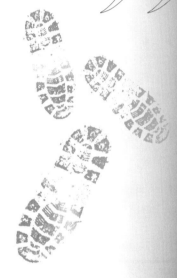

RATINGS

Beauty: ☆ ☆ ☆ ☆ ☆
Privacy: ☆
Spaciousness: ☆ ☆
Quiet: ☆ ☆ ☆
Security: ☆ ☆ ☆ ☆ ☆
Cleanliness: ☆ ☆ ☆ ☆

KEY INFORMATION

ADDRESS: Malibu Creek
State Park
Angeles District,
Malibu Sector
1925 Las Virgenes
Road
Calabasas, CA 91302

OPERATED BY: California State
Parks

INFORMATION: (818) 880-0367;
www.parks.ca.gov

OPEN: Year-round

SITES: 63 tent sites; 4
RV sites

EACH SITE HAS: Picnic table, fire
pits, no hookups

ASSIGNMENT: First come, first
served; reservations
recommended in
summer and on
holidays

REGISTRATION: By park entrance;
reserve by phone,
(800) 444-7275, or
online at
www.reserve
america.com.

FACILITIES: Water, flush toilets,
solar-heated showers
(all accessible to
disabled patrons)

PARKING: By site

FEE: $25 ($20 off-season);
$7.50 nonrefundable
reservation fee

ELEVATION: 500 feet

RESTRICTIONS: *Pets:* On leash only;
in campground only
Fires: Charcoal fires
permitted year-
round; wood fires
may be restricted;
check signs
Alcohol: No
restrictions
Vehicles: RV maxi-
mum length 32 feet
Other: Be careful
with fire.

A good introductory walk is along Shady Trail to Century Lake, then back again. From the campground, walk down to a wide fire road. Cross the stream, and you'll see that the road splits into a high road and a low road. Either one will do. Pass the visitor center and find the Gorge Trail. Follow it upstream to where the creek turns dramatically around volcanic rock cliffs into the Rock Pool. Remember the Tarzan movies and the *Swiss Family Robinson* TV series? Parts from both were filmed here.

Back on the high road, you'll come to the crest of a hill where you can look down on Century Lake. Look around carefully and spot the distinctive hills that doubled for Korean terrain in the television series *M*A*S*H.* When I first hiked the park, part of the set was still lying around, and you could feel the ghosts of Hawkeye, Radar, and all those choppers.

A challenging hike is up to the Backbone Trail. From there, you could conceivably hike all the way to Will Rogers State Park in Los Angeles. Don't try it, though, unless you are a walking fool. Farther on is a swampy pond always good for bird-watching, and then Ronald Reagan's ranch with some good hiking. (Obtain a good map of the park from the ranger at the gate for $1.)

Note that wood fires are only allowed from December to May because of summer fire hazards. This area is near the scene of the 1996 fire that burned down into the heart of Malibu Canyon, wreaking havoc on forests and homes. Fires in the Lower Cha-parral are as common as cats and so much a part of the cycle of nature that Native Americans would set con-trolled fires to help Mother Nature along. They were interested in burning the brush fuel underneath the bigger trees before the brush grew enough to burn the larger trees. Fire also allowed more access and helped expose the game animals.

My favorite time of year here is fall to spring—the park's off-season. I find the mountains too hot in the summer for hiking or biking (pack a canteen if you decide to visit then). However, camping at Malibu Creek State Park in the summer would afford you a

MAP

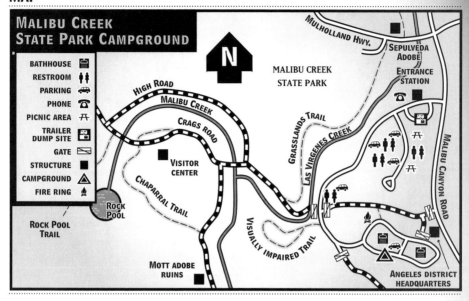

MALIBU CREEK STATE PARK CAMPGROUND

BATHHOUSE	⌂
RESTROOM	♀♂
PARKING	🚗
PHONE	☎
PICNIC AREA	⊼
TRAILER DUMP SITE	▦
GATE	⊠
STRUCTURE	■
CAMPGROUND	△
FIRE RING	♨

MULHOLLAND HWY.

SEPULVEDA ADOBE

MALIBU CREEK STATE PARK

ENTRANCE STATION

HIGH ROAD

MALIBU CREEK

CRAGS ROAD

GRASSLANDS TRAIL

LAS VIRGENES CREEK

MALIBU CANYON ROAD

VISITOR CENTER

CHAPARRAL TRAIL

ROCK POOL

ROCK POOL TRAIL

VISUALLY IMPAIRED TRAIL

MOTT ADOBE RUINS

ANGELES DISTRICT HEADQUARTERS

good base camp to hit the beach and other L.A. summer tourist attractions. Note that the Renaissance Fair is held just up the road at the Paramount Ranch (in Santa Monica Mountains National Recreation Area) along with an old-time western town used in several movies.

GETTING THERE

From Santa Monica, drive north up CA 1 through Malibu, turn right on Malibu Canyon Road, and drive 6 miles to the park entrance on the left. From the San Fernando Valley, drive north on US 101 to the Las Virgenes exit and drive 4 miles southwest on Las Virgenes Road to the park entrance.

GPS COORDINATES

UTM Zone (WGS 84) 11S
Easting 341876
Northing 3774220
Latitude N 34° 5' 49"
Longtitude W 118° 42' 51"

> *In the late summer and early fall, there are few better places on the planet to be. The beach is long, and the water is cool and refreshing.*

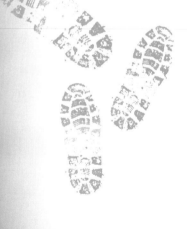

RATINGS

Beauty: ✩ ✩ ✩ ✩
Privacy: ✩ ✩
Spaciousness: ✩ ✩ ✩ ✩
Quiet: ✩ ✩ ✩
Security: ✩ ✩ ✩
Cleanliness: ✩ ✩ ✩ ✩

IN AN UNLIKELY PLACE, McGrath State Beach offers a beach-camping experience unlike any of the others featured in this book. Rather than being situated atop a bluff looking down on the shoreline, or across a highway, the campsites at McGrath State Beach are right on the beach. Although the sand has been replaced with grassy knolls and hard-packed dirt adequate for tents, getting to the beach is a simple trot up and over the small, ice plant–dotted sand drifts, and *presto!* you're looking at a beach utopia you probably didn't know existed, as this stretch of shoreline can't be seen from US 101 or any other oft-traveled route.

McGrath State Beach is a fantastic place to swim and body-surf. The sea bottom has few rocks, if any, and the water doesn't drop off quickly, making McGrath a great place for the kids to play in the water. There's the added factor of being able to beat the crowds—the multitudes know nothing about this beach. An added bonus for some is the lack of alcohol restrictions on the beach and the campsites.

Although McGrath Beach doesn't have a true surf break, the wave composition is similar to what's found at Zuma Beach in Malibu, meaning the waves break randomly along the entire stretch of beach rather that along a singular point or shoal. Nevertheless, the waves are surfable in the right conditions. Windy days are common in the Ventura-Oxnard area, so windsurfing is a possibility too. The 2 miles of coastline are also productive surf-fishing grounds, but there is limited offshore structure to make this place attractive to spear fishermen, kayak fishermen, or scuba divers. Depending on the time of year, surf fishermen can find great bait right beneath their feet as they walk the shoreline pursuing prey. Sand crabs can be found by digging down into the sand, sometimes as little as six inches below the surface. They are candy to all predatory fish in the surf line, and a handful of sand crabs larger than one-half inch in length almost guarantees fishing success. Squid and mussels can also be effective, as are soft plastic jigs. Of course, campers should carry a fishing license at all times and obey fishing regulations.

Perhaps the highlight of McGrath State Beach is the nature trail leading to the Santa Clara River Estuary Natural Preserve. A vigorous effort is under way to restore the lower reaches of the Santa Clara River to their natural state before urban development and to protect the many species of native birds and aquatic life. The Santa Clara River is home to one of the last natural steelhead runs in Southern California. Steelhead are native rainbow trout with a life cycle similar to salmon, in that they spend the early part of their lives in freshwater streams and rivers, then swim into the ocean, then return to spawn. Steelhead are endangered in SoCal, so fishing for them is strictly forbidden. The Santa Clara River watershed is also a bird-watchers paradise, home to many rare and endangered species of birds.

McGrath State Beach is encapsulated by vast plots of farmland. Their very existence in such a seemingly lucrative area is a true oddity. Although the area is famous for its strawberry harvests, many different types of produce can be purchased at the various farmers' markets. Two particularly large markets are very close to McGrath State Beach—to visit them, drive north on Harbor Boulevard for approximately 1.5 miles, then turn right, heading east on Olivas Park Road for approximately 1.25 miles. Two markets are found at this intersection, on both sides of the road, and are a pleasant break from shopping at crowded, annoying supermarkets. While searching for that perfect melon or bag of ripe cherries, ponder why the farmland of the Oxnard-Ventura area hasn't been bought up by developers and transformed into a beachside suburban terror. That it hasn't just doesn't make any sense. Hopefully, the farms will stay forever. Oxnard gives us a taste of what California coastal cities may have looked like before their populations exploded and development swallowed up every shred of available land.

KEY INFORMATION

ADDRESS:	2211 Harbor Blvd. Oxnard, CA 93035; (805) 654-4744
OPERATED BY:	California State Parks
INFORMATION:	(805) 968-1033; www.parks.ca.gov
OPEN:	Year-round
SITES:	173
EACH SITE HAS:	Fire ring, picnic table
ASSIGNMENT:	Reservations can be made online at www.reserve america.com or by calling (800) 444-7275.
REGISTRATION:	Self-registration if park entrance station is closed
FACILITIES:	Showers, running water, bathrooms
PARKING:	On site
FEE:	$25; $20 off-season (Dec. 1–Feb. 28); $7.50 reservation fee
ELEVATION:	Sea level
RESTRICTIONS:	*Pets:* Dogs must be kept on a 6-foot leash at all times, are not permitted on beach or in buildings, and must be inside vehicle or tent at night.

MAP

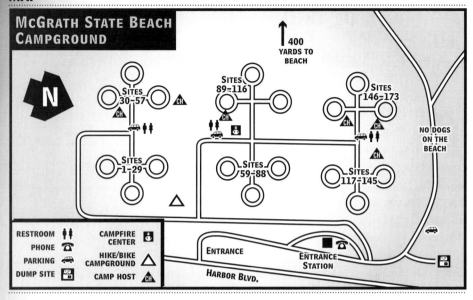

McGrath State Beach Campground

400 YARDS TO BEACH

N

SITES 30–57

SITES 89–116

SITES 146–173

SITES 1–29

SITES 59–88

SITES 117–145

NO DOGS ON THE BEACH

RESTROOM	CAMPFIRE CENTER
PHONE	HIKE/BIKE CAMPGROUND
PARKING	
DUMP SITE	CAMP HOST

ENTRANCE

ENTRANCE STATION

HARBOR BLVD.

GETTING THERE

From central Los Angeles, head north on US 101 approximately 60 miles, exit at South Victoria Avenue, and turn left. After driving 4 miles on Victoria Avenue, turn right on West Fifth Street. After 1.2 miles, turn left on Harbor Boulevard, and in another 1.4 miles the entrance to McGrath State Beach will appear on the right.

The campsites at McGrath State Beach are less spread out and private than those found at other beaches, but they are highly sought-after nonetheless, so booking well in advance is essential. The best sites lie closest to the shoreline, up against the line of sandy bluffs that form a boundary between the park and the beach. McGrath truly keeps it simple—sun, sand, and waves. In the late summer and early fall, there are few better places to be on the planet. The beach is long, and the water is cool and refreshing. Book your sites ASAP.

GPS COORDINATES

UTM Zone (WGS 84) 11S
Easting 292233
Northing 3788950
Latitude N 34° 13' 15"
Longitude W 119° 15' 20"

08
MONTAÑA DE ORO
STATE PARK
CAMPGROUND

AFTER A WEEK, SMOGGY LOS ANGELES seems full of snarling attack dogs and urbanites ready to carve out your liver over a parking space. But drive north of Santa Barbara where the air is clear and you'll see hikers on cliffs at sunset, parents with babies in backpacks, ball-chasing Labrador retrievers, and unattended bicycles—especially at Montaña de Oro State Park. Its rocky azure coves feel like Greece; the sandwiched cliffs jutting out over the ocean remind you of Cornwall; and the long sand dunes resemble Provincetown on the Cape. With 7 miles of spectacular coast, this is one of California's largest state parks.

Montaña de Oro was Chumash Indian territory until the Spanish Mission Period. The Chumash were missionized, then left without a way of life when the missions were secularized. Then came the Pechos, a Spanish family who dealt in cattle, and the ranching Spooners. Then Alexander Hazard planted hundreds of eucalyptus trees here in hopes of selling them to the railroad for ties. Hazard's lumber dreams hit the same rocks as those of other Southern California eucalyptus timber barons. The trees grew fast, but the tree grain spindled, making the tree useless—even as firewood.

Some thought the wrong variety of eucalyptus was imported from Australia, but not so. Botanists have determined that eucalyptus planted in California has no natural pests, so it grows so fast it spindles. In Australia, insects slow trees' growth so their trunks don't spindle.

Today, Montaña de Oro State Park begins at the Morro Rock and goes south along a huge sandspit some 85 feet high. This is a prime area for hiking, picnicking, sunbathing, and swimming. You can get lost in little, private, sandy hollows in the dunes. On one side, you can see the sea, and on the other, Morro Bay, the largest, least-disturbed saltwater marsh in California.

> *Year-round camping with 7 miles of virgin California coast.*

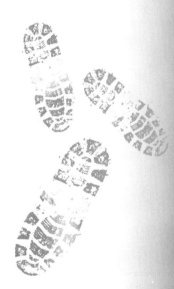

RATINGS

Beauty: ✪ ✪ ✪ ✪ ✪
Privacy: ✪ ✪
Spaciousness: ✪ ✪ ✪
Quiet: ✪ ✪
Security: ✪ ✪ ✪ ✪ ✪
Cleanliness: ✪ ✪ ✪ ✪ ✪

KEY INFORMATION

Bring a big backpack crammed with a blanket, water, food, and sunscreen, because the sandspit is an all-day affair.

Farther south, the sandspit gives way to more dunes that fall off to cliffs, flat sheet rock, and small cove beaches below. Park on Pecho Valley Road above at turnouts and hike over the dune and down. Again, bring supplies, because once you get down there, you won't want to leave.

Finally, from Park Headquarters south is an ancient wave-cut terrace with sharp, upended cliffs of Monterey shale that fall abruptly to the sea. Here and there, you'll spot accessible coves offering more sunbathing and wading (at low tide only). Don't miss Corallina Cove, about a mile south of the Ranch House visitor center. At low tide, you can spot the plants and animals that live in the tidal pools. Obtain a free pamphlet and tidal schedule at the visitor center before you go.

East, off the coast, the park takes in about 8,000 acres of prime hiking, including Valencia Peak at 1,347 feet. From here, you can see the whole sweep of coast from Vandenberg Air Force Base (64 miles) in the south to Piedras Blancas (80 miles) in the north. I think Montaña de Oro provides the best spring hiking in California. By summer, it is too hot.

The two-loop campground is in the canyon just behind Spooner Cove, where big sailing ships once unloaded supplies and took on hides and tallow (for candles). Here, the canyon is narrow and runs along Islay Creek, which Spooner dammed up to run a water wheel for power. All traffic goes by the neck of the canyon. It gets busy, so the best camping is in the back loop. As a trade-off, you'll have a longer walk to the beach from the back. Weekends are busy in the summer, so reserve early.

Camping in the canyon is close, but the atmosphere is friendly. The Ranger Station is right by the headquarters, and the information center is staffed by friendly locals. Montaña de Oro Campground makes you feel warm and safe. In the summer, count on lots of children. This means bicycles, skateboards, in-line skates, and the trill of youthful voices. Montaña de Oro

MAP

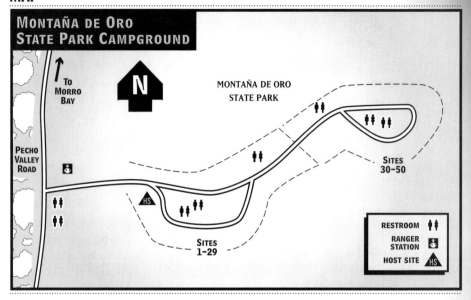

MONTAÑA DE ORO STATE PARK CAMPGROUND

To MORRO BAY

N

MONTAÑA DE ORO STATE PARK

PECHO VALLEY ROAD

SITES 30–50

SITES 1–29

RESTROOM
RANGER STATION
HOST SITE

is a prime family tent camping vacation spot. If you can't handle that, head for the walk-in environmental campsites scattered in the park.

There is tap water; however, it is so heavily chlorinated that it is useful for washing only, so bring drinking water. Also, bring one of those plastic-bag showers to hang in a tree and sluice off the sand and salt. It wouldn't be a bad idea to bring a bucket to set by the tent for dipping sandy feet, and a brush and dust pan to keep sand out of your tent.

GETTING THERE

From L.A., drive north on US 101 to the outskirts of San Luis Obispo. Turn left on Los Osos Valley Road and drive west to Los Osos, where the road becomes Pecho Valley Road. Continue south 5 miles to Montaña de Oro State Park.

GPS COORDINATES

UTM Zone (WGS 84) 10S
Easting 692793
Northing 3905491
Latitude N 35° 16' 26"
Longtitude W 120° 52' 49"

09
PINNACLES
CAMPGROUND

Enjoy easy, hike-in access to Pinnacles National Monument from privately run Pinnacles Campground.

PINNACLES NATIONAL MONUMENT is a fascinating park. Miles of challenging trails thread over rock outcrops, along creeks, and even through caves. Unfortunately, the park's prime walk-in campground, on the west side of the park, was washed away in 1998's El Niño flooding, and there are no plans to rebuild. Fortunately, a wonderful, privately run campground sits just over the park's eastern boundary.

Pinnacles National Monument has limited parking inside the park; by setting up a base camp at the campground, you can walk into the park, or take a convenient shuttle bus. This translates to extra snuggle time in your sleeping bag, because even when the national monument's lots fill early, you won't be turned away on foot. From April to October, cool down after a grueling hike with a dip in the campground pool, then return to your campsite and lounge about.

Most of the campground's sites are at least partly shaded by coast live oaks, and there is a pleasant feeling of spaciousness at this campground. The owners really work on keeping the place clean, quiet, and safe, and the tent sites are all strung together a good distance from the RV and group sites. On summer weekends, park rangers often host programs at the amphitheater, and when we last camped here, the ranger got a good crowd. We stayed at our campsite by the fire, and listened to the ranger teach the kids in the audience how to howl like a coyote.

Camping here is particularly delightful in early spring, when wildflowers are breathtaking and the trails at the national monument are still cool. If you have the stamina for summer hiking on these mostly exposed trails, be sure to bring lots and lots of water, and get an early start. Pinnacles' most famous features are rock formations and caves, and you can get a short

RATINGS

Beauty: ✿ ✿ ✿ ✿
Privacy: ✿ ✿ ✿
Spaciousness: ✿ ✿ ✿
Quiet: ✿ ✿ ✿
Security: ✿ ✿ ✿ ✿ ✿
Cleanliness: ✿ ✿ ✿ ✿ ✿

orientation to both on Bear Gulch Caves Trail, which departs from the Bear Gulch visitor center, or a day-long tour de force on a hike combining Balconies Caves and High Peaks trails. The caves at Bear Gulch are closed for most of the year (to protect a threatened species of bat; call ahead for dates), while Balconies is generally open all year, unless high water floods the cave.

If you can manage it, the longer hike is highly recommended. Start at the campground with one flashlight per person (believe me, you will stretch the bonds of a relationship attempting to share a flashlight), and walk west 1.7 easy miles to a junction with the trail to Bear Gulch on the left and the trail to High Peaks on the right. Continue to the right for 0.6 more miles, then arrive at the Chalone Creek trailhead. Pick your poison: High Peaks is steep and Balconies Caves is nearly level. I like to get to the cave early, so I prefer Balconies Caves, 2.3 miles from this trailhead. From Chalone Creek trailhead, hike west on Old Pinnacles Trail, following close to Chalone Creek, then reaching Balconies Cave. Here, the trail enters Balconies Cave—it's only 0.4 miles to daylight on the other side, but the cave is quite a thrill nonetheless, as you must follow the series of blazes and climb over some talus rocks through utter darkness.

After exiting the cave, blinking, it's another 0.6 miles to the Chaparral Ranger Station at the west side of the park. Be sure to fill up your water, then start to climb on Juniper Canyon Trail, a sharp ascent into the rock formations that give the park its name. From the High Peaks area, you'll likely see vultures and hawks, but also look for California condors, which have been reintroduced to the area. Return to Chalone Creek via High Peaks Trail, then retrace your steps to the campground. Altogether, this hike is 11.5 miles, but the only really hard section is the part from Chaparral, the western trailhead, to Chalone Creek, and if you get an early enough start, you could shave off some miles by driving to the Chalone Creek trailhead.

Climbing is also permitted in the park—call ahead for current conditions and seasonal closures that protect nesting raptors. As you spend time in the park, be alert for wild pigs. When my friend Kelly and I stopped at the

KEY INFORMATION

ADDRESS:	Pinnacles Campground, Inc. 2400 CA 146 Paicines, CA 95043
OPERATED BY:	National Park Service
INFORMATION:	(831) 389-4485; www.nps.gov/pinn
OPEN:	Year-round
SITES:	77 tent-only sites, 36 sites for RVs, 15 tent group sites, 1 RV group site
EACH SITE HAS:	Fire ring, picnic table
ASSIGNMENT:	Site-specific reservations accepted
REGISTRATION:	At store (campground entrance); reserve by phone (877) 444-6777 or online at www.recreation.gov.
FACILITIES:	Flush toilets, drinking water, firewood for sale, swimming pool (seasonal), coin-operated hot showers, store
PARKING:	At site
FEE:	$23, plus $9 reservation fee)
ELEVATION:	About 1,000 feet
RESTRICTIONS:	*Pets:* On leash, in campground only *Fires:* In established pits/rings/grills only; wood fires restricted during much of the year, but artificial logs are permitted. *Alcohol:* No restrictions *Other:* Generators, amplified music, and radios are not permitted.

MAP

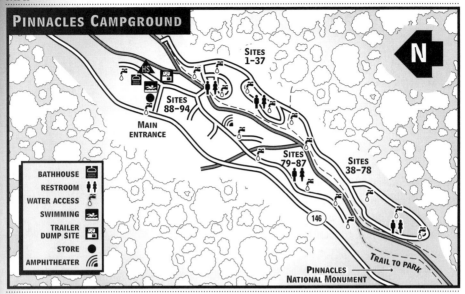

PINNACLES CAMPGROUND

SITES 1-37

SITES 88-94

MAIN ENTRANCE

SITES 79-87

SITES 38-78

146

N

BATHHOUSE	
RESTROOM	
WATER ACCESS	
SWIMMING	
TRAILER DUMP SITE	
STORE	●
AMPHITHEATER	

TRAIL TO PARK

PINNACLES NATIONAL MONUMENT

GETTING THERE

From US 101 in Gilroy, exit CA 25. Drive 13 miles south into Hollister, then follow CA 25 as it weaves through Hollister. Continue 31 miles south on CA 25, then turn right onto CA 146. Drive about 2 miles, then turn left into the campground.

GPS COORDINATES

UTM Zone (WGS84) 10S
Easting 663847
Northing 4040103
Latitude N 36° 29' 32"
Longtitude W 121° 10' 42"

far side of Balconies Cave for a restorative snack, we heard pigs grunting nearby and quickly left the area.

The campground store is small, so stock up in Hollister. In spring and summer you'll likely see fresh produce for sale at farm stands on the road from Gilroy to Hollister, but this rapidly expanding area south of San Jose has many large supermarkets and stores. Garlic is king around Gilroy (the garlic capital of the world), and if you believe that garlic does repel mosquitoes as folk wisdom claims, you can stack the cards in your favor with a plethora of garlic-infused products available at stands and stores along US 101. Once you get to the campground you'll have to drive to the small settlements of Tres Piños and Paicines, about 18 miles north of the park, for a restaurant-cooked meal. South of the campground and park, CA 25 is one of the most scenic drives in the area; this lonely road winds through grassland dotted with ranches, where there are far more cattle than people. I once saw a large herd of elk along the side of CA 25, and it barely made me blink—this part of San Benito County seems to linger with one foot in the past, when grizzly bears roamed the state.

10
POINT MUGU STATE PARK: BIG SYCAMORE CANYON CAMPGROUND

A **SCHOOL OF DOLPHINS PUSHING** bait fish into the shore, working them around the rocky points—dolphin skin wet black against the blue water—that was my first impression of Point Mugu State Park's Big Sycamore Canyon Campground. The beach is gorgeous, a white-sand jewel of a place to picnic, sun, and swim on an unspoiled stretch of coastline.

Just outside Los Angeles, Point Mugu State Park is a jewel.

Later, I discovered that the Chumash Native Americans once lived in the canyon and believed that dolphins were their brothers. At one time, the Chumash lived on overpopulated islands to the west. Legend has it that their mother god told them to cross over the sea to the mainland by walking on a rainbow. The caveat was that they couldn't look down. Of course, some did and fell into the sea. But, the mother god took pity on them and turned them into dolphins.

The Chumash fished from canoes 25 feet long, lashed with sinew and caulked with asphalt from seeps. They gathered clams, oysters, and abalone along the shores and made soapstone bows inlaid with mother-of-pearl from the shells. They hunted and gathered food in the upper reaches of the canyon and lived a life of ease, culture, and bounty. However, the Spanish put a quick end to that, and now we can camp where the Chumash lived at the mouth of the canyon, where it is cool in the summer and warm in the winter.

Like Malibu Creek State Park, Point Mugu State Park and Big Sycamore Canyon Campground are heavily used, both for overnight camping and for day use. Buses of schoolkids come for the morning. Mountain bikers access the fire roads up in the canyon. And many hikers come for the wildflowers. Still, the pristine beaches, rolling hills, savanna meadows, and the glorious canyon so close to the Greater Los Angeles Metropolitan Area make Big Sycamore Canyon a must-visit campground. Try to visit in the off-season,

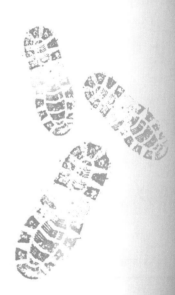

RATINGS

Beauty: ✪ ✪ ✪ ✪ ✪
Privacy: ✪ ✪
Spaciousness: ✪ ✪ ✪
Quiet: ✪ ✪ ✪
Security: ✪ ✪ ✪ ✪ ✪
Cleanliness: ✪ ✪ ✪ ✪ ✪

ADDRESS: Big Sycamore
Canyon
Campground
Point Mugu State
Park
Angeles District
1925 Las Virgenes
Road
Calabasas, CA 91302

OPERATED BY: California State
Parks

INFORMATION: (818) 488-5223,
www.parks.ca.gov

OPEN: Year-round

SITES: 58

EACH SITE HAS: Picnic tables, fire
grills

ASSIGNMENT: First come, first
served; reservations
recommended in
summer

REGISTRATION: At entrance; reserve
by phone, (800)
444-7275, or online,
www.reserve
america.com.

FACILITIES: Water, flush toilets,
coin-operated
showers

PARKING: At site

FEE: $25 ($20 off-season);
$7.50 nonrefundable
reservation fee

ELEVATION: Sea level

RESTRICTIONS: *Pets:* Dogs allowed
on leash in
campground only,
not on trails
Fires: Allowed (no
wood gathering)
Alcohol: No
restrictions
Vehicles: RVs up to
31 feet

but watch the weather to schedule the best hiking days. Or, reserve ahead and hit the beach in the summer. The canyon is cool enough in summer for biking. Prime surf fishing is available off Thornhill Broome Beach, just up the road.

This is an excellent area for viewing monarch butterflies. They clump in the sycamore in the canyon and eat milkweed up in the meadows. Why don't sea gulls descend on the easily spotted, brightly decorated monarchs and have a big chow-down? Because milkweed is poisonous. Rasputin used it to knock off members of the Russian court. Milkweed is toxic enough so that when birds pick up a milkweed-eating monarch, they feel sick and learn to leave them alone. The monarch's bright colors serve to alert the birds to eat at their own risk.

In Big Sycamore Canyon, you'll find many sycamores. You'll also find coast live oak and areas of chaparral and coastal shrub. Look for blue elderberry, wild rose, California bay, purple sage, and, of course, poison oak. Make a habit of washing your hands and other exposed areas with dish detergent after a hike, and don't swim in any stream or stream-fed pond after even a gentle rain. The oil from the poison oak gets in the water and will make you very unhappy.

Like Malibu Creek State Park, there is a Ranger Headquarters at Point Mugu State Park, near Big Sycamore Campground. The park feels safe, well regulated, and well patrolled, which is comforting so close to dense urban areas. If you tire of Point Mugu's small beach, remember there are miles of beaches just a short drive away. Neptune's Net, just south of the campground, is a good place to eat fish-and-chips or buy crab or lobster to grill. On some weekends, the outdoor patio restaurant can be overrun with biker gangs. Of course, upon close examination, the bikers look and act like very well-behaved middle-class Americans (and probably are!). They fit right in with the younger surfers and middle-aged campers.

You must plan a visit to Point Mugu and Big Sycamore Canyon. Watch the weather and avoid the June blahs. Beware of weather predictions calling for "early-morning and late-afternoon fog along the

MAP

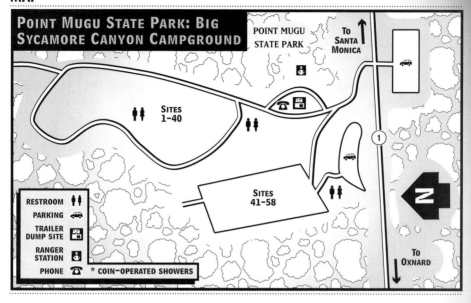

POINT MUGU STATE PARK: BIG
SYCAMORE CANYON CAMPGROUND

POINT MUGU
STATE PARK

To
SANTA
MONICA

SITES
1–40

SITES
41–58

RESTROOM
PARKING
TRAILER
DUMP SITE
RANGER
STATION
PHONE   * COIN-OPERATED SHOWERS

1

N

To
OXNARD

coastline." And don't forget to make reservations.
Don't expect the campground itself to be too scenic.
Look to the sea, the sky, and the canyon for incredi-
ble vistas.

GETTING THERE

From L.A., drive 32 miles
north up CA 1 or drive
16 miles south from Oxnard.

GPS COORDINATES

UTM Zone (WGS 84) 11S
Easting 314095
Northing 3772091
Latitude N 34° 4' 23"
Longtitude W 119° 0' 53"

REYES CREEK CAMPGROUND

> *This campground is dominated by Reyes Creek—every site is either creekside or nearby.*

IS THERE ANY SLEEP AID** more potent than a rushing stream? The sound of rushing water always puts me to sleep and keeps me there throughout the night, and that's exactly what happened at Reyes Creek. Even though we were camped a good distance from the water, the murmur of the creek provided the perfect volume of white noise for peaceful sleeping.

This campground is open all year and features generously spaced sites on and near the creek, where you can fish for rainbow trout or splash about in hot weather. Set in a wide, shallow bowl, the campground is dominated by scrub oak, manzanita, pinyon pine, chamise, silktassel, and, near the creek, live oak, cottonwood, and alder. Small boulders and sandstone formations are prominent in the surrounding low, chaparral-studded hills. At just less than 4,000 feet, Reyes Creek Campground is best suited to spring and autumn camping, although there is a substantial amount of tree cover to shade you during the dusty months of summer, when a dip in the creek is just about mandatory. When we camped here in late April, the sites along the creek were full, but we were the only campers in the campground's largest loop, where a grassy, open meadow in the middle of the sites is perfect for soaking up some sun in the afternoon. During the day the temperature was perfect, but it got s eriously chilly once the sun dropped, and we ate breakfast while trying to keep our hands tucked in our jacket pockets. During the afternoon, a breeze rustled through the campground's pinyon pines, cottontail rabbits munched in the underbrush, and humming-birds zipped around searching for nectar.

This is an old campground (Camp Scheideck dates from the 1890s) that feels slightly shabby (in a National Forest kind of way); some of the picnic tables

RATINGS

Beauty: ✩ ✩ ✩ ✩
Privacy: ✩ ✩ ✩
Spaciousness: ✩ ✩ ✩
Quiet: ✩ ✩ ✩
Security: ✩ ✩
Cleanliness: ✩ ✩ ✩

look like they were installed during the Kennedy administration. Just a few pieces of garbage strewn about a campsite can really make the area feel more run-down than it is, and I always volunteer a little light housekeeping before we pack up and leave any campsite. It usually takes only minutes to pick up any bottle caps and stray pieces of garbage, and I think that when campers arrive at a clean site, most are more likely to leave the site clean.

If you aren't content to fish or relax in your campsite, you can hike right from the campground. A short, paved, dead-end spur departs from the campground to the trailhead for Gene Marshall-Piedra Blanca Trail, a narrow footpath running 17 miles southeast through Sespe Wilderness, passing a string of backcountry campsites before ending at Lion Campground. A few hours of out-and-back hiking on this trail earns an afternoon nap for sure.

Reyes Creek campground is adjacent to a funky and rustic private camp, which sells ice and even cocktails, but for more substantial supplies, shop in Ojai—there are no other settlements in this area.

"Semi-primitive" campgrounds are plentiful in this part of Los Padres National Forest, where campground elevations range from around 2,000 feet (Wheeler Gorge) to 7,800 feet (Mount Pinos). There are numerous other camping options within a 20-mile radius of Reyes Creek, most of which are small, nonreservable campgrounds with pit toilets, picnic tables, and fire rings, but no water. The campgrounds at the higher elevations, including Reyes Peak and Mount Piños, are closed in winter, but two of Reyes Creek's nearest neighbors, Ozena and Pine Springs, are open year-round. On the way from Ojai, check out Rose Valley Campground on Sespe River Road, nine sites only 0.6 miles from Rose Valley Falls, or Reyes Peak Campground, six sites at 6,800 feet, a cooler summer choice. With the Los Padres National Forest map in hand you could scout all these campgrounds, settling for your favorite; if you live in Santa Barbara or greater Los Angeles, Reyes Creek and the other nearby campgrounds may quickly become your regular destination

KEY INFORMATION

ADDRESS: Mount Piños Ranger District
Los Padres National Forest
34580 Lockwood Valley Road
Frazier Park, CA 93225

OPERATED BY: Los Padres National Forest

INFORMATION: (805) 968-6640; www.fs.fed.us/r5/lospadres

OPEN: Year-round

SITES: 30 sites for tents and RVs

EACH SITE HAS: Fire ring, picnic table

ASSIGNMENT: First come, first served; no reservations

REGISTRATION: Obtain a National Forest Adventure Pass in advance, available at locations throughout the forest, or by mail: San Bernardino National Forest, Fee Project Headquarters, 1824 South Commercenter Circle, San Bernardino, CA 92408. In Ojai, you can pick one up at the Ojai Ranger District, 1190 East Ojai Ave., Ojai 93023; (805) 646-4348.

FACILITIES: Pit toilets

PARKING: At site

FEE: $5 (Adventure Pass)

ELEVATION: 3,960 feet

RESTRICTIONS: *Pets:* On leash
Fires: In established pits/rings only; may be prohibited during high fire danger
Alcohol: No restrictions

MAP

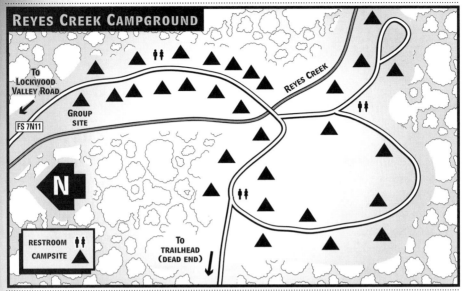

REYES CREEK CAMPGROUND

To
LOCKWOOD
VALLEY ROAD

FS 7N11

GROUP
SITE

REYES CREEK

N

RESTROOM
CAMPSITE

To
TRAILHEAD
(DEAD END)

GETTING THERE

From Ojai, drive north on CA 33 for 36 miles, turn right onto Lockwood Valley Road, drive 3.2 miles, then turn right onto FS 7N11, signed to Reyes Creek Campground. Continue another 1.5 miles, past Scheideck Camp and Lodge, to the campground.

to escape summer heat. Be sure to use extra caution with your campfires here, particularly in summer and autumn, when the surrounding forest is dry and prone to wildfires. Although open all year, Lockwood Valley Road and the road to the campground cross washes and may be impassable during wet weather—call ahead to check, and don't forget to bring your own water.

GPS COORDINATES

UTM Zone (WGS 84) 11S
Easting 288506
Northing 3839877
Latitude N 34° 40' 45"
Longtitude W 119° 18' 31"

12
THORNHILL BROOME BEACH CAMPGROUND

THORNHILL BROOME BEACH campgrounds are the only ones in SoCal that permit camping right down to the water line, which means you can set up your tent anywhere on the beach, unlike at McGrath or El Capitan, which only allow camping within sites above or behind the actual beach. The attraction of Thornhill Broome's genuine beach camping more than justifies the six-month waiting period needed to book one of the 68 sites during peak season.

From a geographic perspective, Thornhill Broome Beach lies between two points—Point Mugu to the northeast and a small point west of Sycamore Cove—and spans roughly 1.5 miles. The beach is rocky and the surf is usually very rough and exposed to open ocean swells, so swimming is advisable for experienced swimmers only on all but the flattest of days. At the southeast end, opposite the ocean and across CA 1 (the Pacific Coast Highway), is a large sand dune. The northwest end terminates into Point Mugu, which features a large rocky formation. Just southeast of point Mugu and across CA 1 lies the entrance to La Jolla Canyon and the vast network of trails heading into the Santa Monica Mountains and Point Mugu State Park.

There's lots to do at Thornhill Broome Beach aside from typical beach activities like sunbathing and swimming (with caution, of course). Hiking types will be pleased to know they're privy to many miles of trails accessible via La Jolla Canyon. Hard-core mountain bikers have easy access to the trail networks of neighboring Big Sycamore Canyon. Surf fishermen can try their luck at the California Halibut, Corbina, and Surf Perch teeming in the rough waters, and windsurfers will be pleased to find more than satisfactory conditions most of the year. Surfers and divers, on the other hand, will find little of interest at this locale and would be much happier at Leo Carrillo.

> *Thornhill Broome Beach campgrounds are the only ones in SoCal that permit camping right down to the water line.*

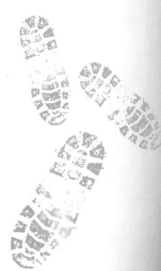

RATINGS

Beauty: ✪ ✪ ✪ ✪ ✪
Privacy: ✪ ✪
Spaciousness: ✪ ✪ ✪ ✪ ✪
Quiet: ✪ ✪
Security: ✪ ✪ ✪
Cleanliness: ✪ ✪ ✪ ✪

ADDRESS:	9000 West Pacific Coast Highway Malibu, CA 90265
OPERATED BY:	Califonia State Parks
INFORMATION:	www.parks.ca.gov/ default.asp?page_id =630
OPEN:	Year-round
SITES:	68
EACH SITE:	Picnic table, fire ring
ASSIGNMENT:	Reservations can be made online at www.reserve america.com or by calling (800) 444-7275.
REGISTRATION:	Self-registration if park entrance station is closed
PARKING:	No day use permitted; $4 parking fee for extra vehicles
FACILITIES:	Toilets, running water, one cold-water shower
FEE:	$15; $11 off-season (Dec. 1–Feb. 28); $7.50 reservation fee
ELEVATION:	Sea level
RESTRICTIONS:	*Pets:* Dogs should be kept on a leash at all times and inside tents or vehicles at night. Glass bottles are prohibited. *Fires:* Permitted inside established fire rings *Alcohol:* No restrictions

Though it's somewhat of a long shot, catching a keeper-sized halibut from shore at Thornhill Broome beach can happen, but certain times of year are better than others. In the spring, the largest numbers of halibut enter shallow waters accessible to surf fishermeen. Though these fish can be caught with bait, experienced anglers prefer casting artificial lures to cover the most area. A licensed fisherman may take no halibut smaller than 22 inches in length. Taking undersized fish and/or fishing without a fishing license is an offense that carries serious penalties, so please play by the rules.

On really clear days, it's possible to see as many as four islands offshore in the horizon, but most days Anacapa Island, the smallest of the Channel Islands archipelago, will be visible to the west, just behind which lies Santa Cruz Island. If the air is pristine, a small blip of land can be visible to the south. Easily confused with distant tanker ships, Santa Barbara Island is a lonely rock located more than 40 miles south of Thornhill Broome Beach. Seeing Catalina Island to the Southeast is unlikely, but it is possible. Seeing the Channel Islands to the west is an enlightening experience for many—too many people in Los Angeles believe Santa Catalina is the only island near shore in the vicinity of SoCal. In fact, there are eight islands in all, Santa Cruz being the largest.

As idyllic as Thornhill Broome seems on paper, there are some downsides. The shoreline is more exposed to wind and high seas than most beaches in SoCal, meaning it can be pretty cold even when it's hot everywhere else. The waters aren't very inviting year-round, due to constant riptides and low water temperatures, so amphibious folk won't be very happy. The trails at La Jolla Canyon and Big Sycamore are fantastic, but crossing the Pacific Coast Highway can be very dangerous, with no crosswalks available and cars roaring by at 60-plus miles per hour. The highway is also a source of constant noise, which can interfere with tranquility.

Campers needn't be choosy about site selection, because each of the 68 sites is smack-dab on the shoreline. If you intend to swim, pick a site between 1 and 10, as they are closest to the lone lifeguard tower. If

MAP

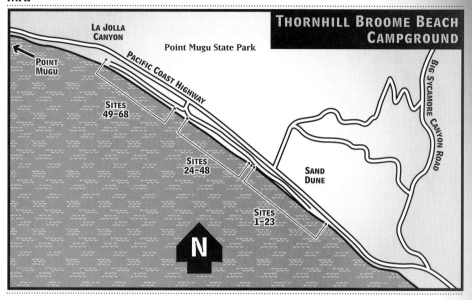

THORNHILL BROOME BEACH CAMPGROUND

La Jolla Canyon

Point Mugu State Park

Point Mugu

Pacific Coast Highway

Sites 49–68

Sites 24–48

Sites 1–23

Sand Dune

Big Sycamore Canyon Road

N

you want easy access to La Jolla Canyon, a higher-numbered site is best, and the opposite is true for mountain bikers, because Big Sycamore Canyon is located around the point to the southeast.

All in all, Thornhill Broome may be the most genuine beach-camping experience north of Baja California. Sadly, you'll have to be very forward-thinking to enjoy this place because of the six-month waiting period and the fact that rangers wait until very late to cancel reservations for no-shows. For sure, Thornhill Broome Beach is beautiful and worthy of any hassle.

GETTING THERE

From Los Angeles, drive east on Interstate 10 until it ends and becomes CA 1, or Pacific Coast Highway. Driving west, stay on CA 1 for 32.7 miles until you reach Big Sycamore Canyon on the right, beyond Malibu. Thornhill Broome Beach is just around the corner, starting roughly 0.25 miles west of Sycamore Cove.

GPS COORDINATES

UTM Zone (WGS 84) 11S
Easting 312406
Northing 3773095
Latitude N 34° 04' 55"
Longitude W 119° 01' 59"

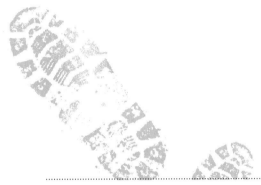
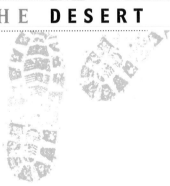

THE **DESERT**

13
ARROYO SALADO PRIMITIVE CAMPGROUND

ARROYO **S**ALADO **IS BADLANDS** camping. It is in malpais (badlands) in the huge Anza-Borrego Desert State Park (ABDSP), which has everything—palm-studded canyons, cactus gardens, mountain pinyon forests, hot springs, waterfalls, bighorn sheep, Native American pictographs and petroglyphs, historic settler trails, stage stops, and ghost towns. A good way to come into Arroyo Salado is on CA 86, off I-10, via Indio and Coachella through the date palm orchards. Stop and have a date shake at one of the stands. Then, carry on along the shore past Salton City Beach and turn east on S-22. Notice Travertine Point on the right and the wave terraces cut into the mountainsides—in recent geological times, the Salton basin was a huge lake. Near the wave terraces are traces of the Native Americans who lived by the lake.

Now, you're in the malpais. This area is characterized by abrupt gullies with banks of sun-hardened clay, gravel-strewn sand, and strange shapes of clay. Red and yellow are the prevailing colors, with mud-hued grays and drabs for a background. After the winter rains, all the flowers bloom—flame-tipped ocotillo, verbena, desert sunflower, lavender, brittlebush, creosote bush, primrose, teddy-bear cholla, and beavertail cactus. The entrance to the Arroyo Salado primitive camping area is 11.8 miles on the left (or, from the opposite direction, 19 miles from the Park headquarters in Borrego Springs). The campground is marked by a metal sign reading "Arroyo Salado." As with all the signs in ABDSP, it is small and unannounced, so you have to be on your toes to see it. There is a turnaround past the entrance to make re-approaching a little easier.

An often-sandy road goes down the wash with various turnoffs where you can park your car and

> *Situated in malpais (badlands) with lizards, flowers, and the rainbow colors of the dunes.*

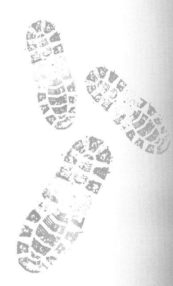

RATINGS

Beauty: ✪ ✪ ✪ ✪ ✪
Privacy: ✪ ✪ ✪ ✪ ✪
Spaciousness: ✪ ✪ ✪ ✪ ✪
Quiet: ✪ ✪ ✪ ✪ ✪
Security: ✪
Cleanliness: ✪ ✪ ✪ ✪

ADDRESS:	Arroyo Salado Primitive Campground Anza-Borrego Desert State Park 200 Palm Canyon Dr. Borrego Springs, CA 92004
OPERATED BY:	California State Parks
INFORMATION:	(760) 767-5311, www.parks.ca.gov
OPEN:	Year-round (avoid summer)
SITES:	Open area
EACH SITE HAS:	No facilities
ASSIGNMENT:	First come, first served; no reservations
REGISTRATION:	Not required
FACILITIES:	Vault toilet; bring plenty of water
PARKING:	Some pullouts; otherwise, less than 10 feet off established dirt roads
FEE:	None
ELEVATION:	880 feet
RESTRICTIONS:	*Pets:* On 6-foot maximum leash; not allowed on trails or in wilderness *Fires:* Only in existing fire rings, or in completely contained metal barbecues; must pack out ashes *Alcohol:* No restrictions *Vehicles:* Suited for pickup campers *Other:* Don't camp near water holes—wildlife depends on them for water; all vegetation (even dead wood) is protected.

camp. Carry your tent up over the hummocks, and, suddenly, you'll be alone in untracked malpais. Everywhere is a good place to pitch a tent. The desert floor is clean and sandy. Sit down and listen to the wind, and look for lizards flitting over the rocks and dunes. Wait, and the desert comes to you.

The road continues down to Seventeen Palms Oasis, Una Palma, and Five Palms. None of these places has the number of palms their names advertise, but there is a spring at Seventeen Palms, as well as a visitor's register consisting of a wooden keg full of notes lodged in the palm fronds of two adjoining palm trees. This desert post office was begun by early-day travelers and prospectors. These considerate travelers also left a fresh water supply for those who followed. The saline water here is drinkable, although highly laxative. In the early 1900s, the famous British traveler J. Smeaton Chase came this way, noting of the water:

> *Rice boiled in it was thoroughly disgusting in color and taste; no amount of sugar could render it more than just bearable. The tea had a dirty gray curdle and a flavor like bilge, and when I tried cocoa as an alternative the mixture promptly went black.*

Past Seventeen Palms, the road continues south and connects with a network of roads in the Borrego Badlands. Don't go any farther unless you have a four-wheel-drive vehicle in good shape, and lots of water. You can camp anywhere you want in ABDSP as long as you don't park more than ten feet off established dirt roads. Of course, you must carry out your garbage. However, a vault toilet spares campers the task of burying waste. No fires are allowed, unless you bring in wood and burn it in a fire ring or a metal container—a portable barbecue would be fine.

Remember, carry a lot of water; one gallon per day, per person should do it. It's not a bad idea to carry a collapsible shovel or sawed-off gardening shovel. If you get stuck in sand, it will be your best friend. Bring some old sheets and light rope. You can sit on one sheet and rig another for shade using the rope. Sleep under a sheet early in the night and get in your sleeping bag later when it gets cold.

MAP

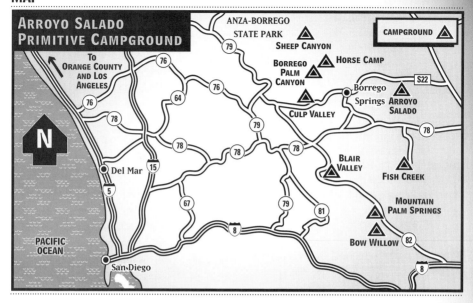

To resupply or to escape the heat, go to Borrego Springs, where vendors sell grapefruit and oranges under shade trees on the traffic circle. Just up Palm Canyon Drive is the visitor center, where you can buy maps and books, and see exhibits. There is an easy 3-mile round-trip nature trail up Borrego Palm Canyon leaving from the Palm Canyon Campground 1 mile from the visitor center. Enjoy the park's more than 400,000 desert acres.

GETTING THERE

From L.A., take I-10 east to CA 86. Head south to the junction with S-22. Turn right and travel 11.8 miles to the entrance on the left. Or, take I-10 east to I-15 south to Temecula. Take CA 79 to the junction with S-2. Take S-2 to S-22 to Borrego Springs. Drive 19 miles east of the visitor center on S-22.

GPS COORDINATES

UTM Zone (WGS84) 11S
Easting 579287
Northing 3682732
Latitude N 33° 16' 51"
Longtitude W 116° 05' 55"

14
LA JOLLA VALLEY
HIKE-IN
CAMPGROUNDS

> *The sites offer 360-degree views without any sign of civilization.*

THE LA JOLLA VALLEY HIKE-IN tent-camping sites are little known and seldom used. Little info about these campsites can be found anywhere, and you may not believe they exist until you motivate yourself to walk up there and take a look. There are a variety of routes to this destination, all of which offer great views of the ocean amid pristine terrain. The number-one reason to visit this place: this is the only true backcountry campground in the Santa Monica Mountains. The sites offer 360-degree views without any sign of civilization, and you'll be hard-pressed to find another soul in the area.

For hikers, there are three logical routes to the La Jolla Valley area. With any of these routes, the objective is to reach La Jolla Valley fire road within the relatively small La Jolla Valley. Hikers coming from Ventura County may want to try the Chumash Trail, which leads directly to the campgrounds in a mostly northeasterly direction. Hikers from the Los Angeles area can make the trek via La Jolla Canyon Trail or by way of Ray Miller Trail. La Jolla Canyon Trail leads almost directly to the sites, ending at La Jolla Valley Fire Road after roughly 2.5 miles, after which one would turn left and walk 0.3 miles, then look for the trails leading to the campgrounds on the right (north) side of the trail. Ray Miller Trail is the least direct, leading to a left turn on Overlook Trail followed by another left on La Jolla Valley fire road, which leads to the campgrounds on the north side after 0.5 miles. Both routes are day hikes and suitable for neophytes because the trails have no major rechnical challenges. It can be very hot, so it's essential to bring as much water as you can carry. Trail maps are available at the ranger kiosks of Big Sycamore Canyon and Thornhill Broome Beach.

You can also bike to La Jolla Valley if you enter

RATINGS

Beauty: ✿ ✿ ✿ ✿
Privacy: ✿ ✿ ✿ ✿ ✿
Spaciousness: ✿ ✿ ✿
Quiet: ✿ ✿ ✿ ✿ ✿
Security: ✿ ✿ ✿ ✿ ✿
Cleanliness: ✿ ✿ ✿ ✿ ✿

via Big Sycamore Canyon-to-Overlook Trail. This is highly recommended if you are able to carry camping gear on your mountain bike. Mountain biking is prohibited everywhere in La Jolla Valley except La Jolla Valley fire road, so walk your bike to the sites and stay off any single-tracks in the area no matter how much you're tempted.

Traveling to the sites may be the most appealing part of the tent-camping experience here. There's nothing like the peace and tranquility of Point Mugu State Park, and the refreshing sea breeze continually brought forth by the Pacific Ocean. This is prime Santa Monica Mountains chaparral scenery, so take it all in as you make the journey. Look for red-tailed hawks, bobcats, rattlesnakes, and deer along the way, and remember that your surroundings are a fine replica of the sites seen by the earliest European explorers of the Southern California region.

It's impossible to visit these secluded sites and not wonder who frequented these areas before Europeans. The Chumash tribe of Native Americans made their home in the Santa Monica Mountains and other parts of SoCal. It's tough to imagine how they secured enough food to survive in such a dry, hot environment, and the answer lies within the oak acorn. The Chumash relied on the acorn as their vegetative staple, supplementing their diets with fish, sea mammals, and birds and land mammals, as well as other native plants. Because hunting in the Santa Monica Mountains is illegal, you'll have to survive on whatever food you packed in.

The trail that leads to the five tent sites (numbered 5 through 9) is a few steps west of the larger group camping sites. The entrance is marked with a small sign that reads "La Jolla Valley Trail Camp"; it leads to a chemical toilet, beyond which are sites 5 through 9 on either side of a narrow trail heading in a northward direction. Along the trail are a few nonfunctional water spigots. There are no trash receptacles, so you'll have to carry everything out. Please don't leave a trace—this is a very special place.

The sites feel very secluded because each has its own narrow, single-track "driveway" leading to a space

KEY INFORMATION

ADDRESS:	9000 West Pacific Coast Highway, Malibu, CA 90265
OPERATED BY:	California State Parks
INFORMATION:	(818) 880-0350; www.nps.gov/samo/ planyourvisit/ camping2.htm
OPEN:	Year-round
SITES:	5
EACH SITE:	Picnic table
ASSIGNMENT:	First come, first served
REGISTRATION:	Self-registration by iron ranger at La Jolla Canyon park entrance
FACILITIES:	Chemical toilets, no running water, trash must be packed out
PARKING:	$10 per day at Big Sycamore Canyon, $4 per day at La Jolla Canyon
FEE:	$3
ELEVATION:	711 feet
RESTRICTIONS:	*Pets:* Not allowed *Fires:* Prohibited at all times *Alcohol:* No restrictions

MAP

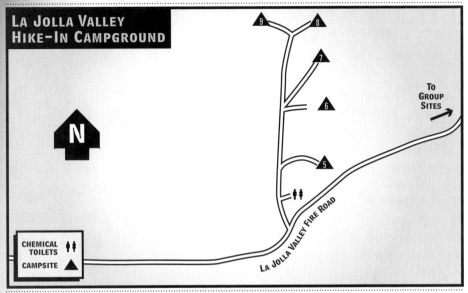

LA JOLLA VALLEY HIKE-IN CAMPGROUND

N

To GROUP SITES →

9 8 7 6 5

La Jolla Valley Fire Road

CHEMICAL TOILETS

CAMPSITE

GETTING THERE

From Los Angeles, drive east on Interstate 10 until it ends and becomes CA 1, or Pacific Coast Highway. Driving west, stay on CA 1 32.7 miles until you reach Big Sycamore Canyon on the right, beyond Malibu. La Jolla Canyon is 1.75 miles farther, also on the right.

GPS COORDINATES

UTM Zone (WGS 84) 11S
Easting 312186
Northing 3775949
Latitude N 34° 06' 27"
Longitude W 119° 02' 10"

carved out of the dense foliage and containing one picnic table and just enough space for a tent or two. Due to the denseness of the vegetation, each site seems totally isolated because the other sites cannot be seen from any vantage point. You may see makeshift fire rings or evidence of campfires, but don't make a fire under any circumstances—you're surrounded by acres of dry, combustible tinder, and fires are strictly prohibited.

Once you've settled in, you can appreciate the peace and remoteness of the area. There are no other legal ways to spend the night in the Santa Monica Mountains. You may, in fact, be spooked by the wildness and seclusion. The La Jolla Valley hike-in campsites are for nature lovers who crave solitude and really want to get away. The experience isn't available anywhere else in the Santa Monica Mountains—it's definitely worthwhile.

15
LITTLE BLAIR VALLEY PRIMITIVE CAMPGROUND

IN THE MIDDLE OF **MARCH,** I camped in Little Blair Valley on the edge of a tremendous meadow. The moon was so full that the tiny flowers sparkled from between the startlingly green grass. What a night!

I was alone until morning when a couple drove by in a rental car. They were lost and looking for the Native American pictographs. We consulted his map, then they were off in a cloud of dust. The rest of the morning it was just me, watching the sun move across the valley and rocks.

The S-2 turnoff to Little Blair Valley is 4 miles south of Scissors Crossing, about 31 miles from ABDSP headquarters in Borrego Springs. On the left, you'll see the tiny stake sign embossed with "Little Blair." The road, usually passable by all passenger cars, goes a mile or so over a ridge into the valley. Here, you'll encounter another stake sign indicating the S-2 highway from which you just came. To the left is a wonderful area for camping in the soft meadow grass.

The road to the right of the S-2 marker curls around the edge of the valley, passing several turnouts with many promising spots for parking and camping. Before you pick one, think about how the sun will travel and when you want to be in the shade or sun.

From here, three short, fun hikes are within easy range. Drive up to the head of Little Blair Valley and you'll see another stake signing the Morteros. There is a parking area and a short 0.75-mile trail leading to large rocks filled with Native American grinding holes. With these *morteros* (mortars), women pulverized coarse seeds and pods, such as mesquite beans, and made a pulp to be dried in the sun and used later for bread. Also, fine seeds and delicate plant parts were rubbed or lightly ground on smooth, polished patches

> *Here you'll find primitive tent camping in a valley full of wildflowers, Native American pictographs, and mortars.*

RATINGS

Beauty: ✿ ✿ ✿ ✿ ✿
Privacy: ✿ ✿ ✿ ✿ ✿
Spaciousness: ✿ ✿ ✿ ✿ ✿
Quiet: ✿ ✿ ✿ ✿ ✿
Security: ✿ ✿
Cleanliness: ✿ ✿ ✿ ✿ ✿

KEY INFORMATION

of rock, known as slicks. The trail continues another mile or so east through a ruggedly beautiful canyon.

From the Morteros parking lot, you can also follow a sign 0.1 mile to the Pictograph Trail. Usually passable, the 1.5-mile dirt road leads to the Pictograph parking lot. From there, climb a ridge and go down the other side to a huge boulder painted in geometric red-and-yellow designs. Notice the different vegetation— juniper, white sage, and pinyon pine.

Go past the pictographs and see more Native American morteros at the base of the ridge to the right. Continue down the wash and into Smuggler Canyon. When the canyon makes a sharp turn to the right, you'll see the Vallecito Valley and the Vallecito Stage Station from the edge of a steep drop.

Smuggler Canyon got its name from the Chinese laborers who came by boat from China, via the Sea of Cortez, to Mexicali. They were then smuggled up to the canyon to avoid law enforcement and angry locals. Once past the frontier, they worked in mines and on farms and railroads. A strenuous hike down Smuggler Canyon will lead you to S-2, a few hundred yards east of Vallecito Stage Station. Arrange a pickup there, since the return is heavy going.

Drive 2 miles past the Morteros pullout into the Blair Valley (not Little Blair Valley), and you'll see a signed turn to the left going to the Marshall South Home on Ghost Mountain. Park in the lot just down the road and hike 1 mile straight up the mountain to see the ruins of the house.

In 1932, Marshall South and his wife, Tanya, built a house on top of the beautiful Ghost Mountain, which they called "Yaquitepec." They saved rainwater in cisterns and ate yucca and agave like the local Native Americans. Supplies were brought in by Model T from the town of Julian and carried up the mountain by mule or man. Marshall and Tanya raised three children and supported themselves by writing for *Desert* magazine. Finally, in a phrase that sends a chill down the spine of every married man, Tanya "tired of the eccentricities of her husband" and moved to San Diego, where she remarried.

MAP

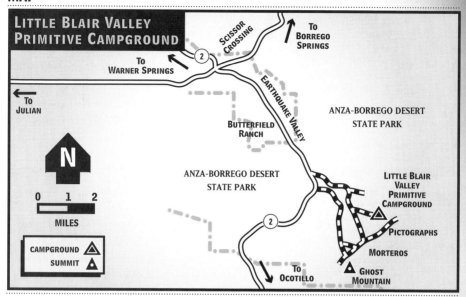

LITTLE BLAIR VALLEY
PRIMITIVE CAMPGROUND

SCISSOR CROSSING

To BORREGO SPRINGS

2

To WARNER SPRINGS

EARTHQUAKE VALLEY

To JULIAN

ANZA-BORREGO DESERT STATE PARK

N

BUTTERFIELD RANCH

ANZA-BORREGO DESERT STATE PARK

LITTLE BLAIR VALLEY PRIMITIVE CAMPGROUND

0   1   2

MILES

CAMPGROUND

SUMMIT

2

PICTOGRAPHS

MORTEROS

To OCOTILLO

GHOST MOUNTAIN

From the parking lot, you can drive back to S-2 through Blair Valley, passing several pullouts and some good camping sites. Blair Valley is regularly trafficked by RVs and tent campers. However, it is a good idea to check with the ABDSP headquarters on the condition of the roads, especially after a rain.

GETTING THERE

From L.A., take I-10 east to I-15. Go south to Temecula. Take CA 79 east past Warner Springs to Julian. From Julian on CA 79, drive 12 miles east to S-2. Go right 4 miles on S-2 and find the stake marker "Little Blair" on the left. Follow the dirt road about a mile to Little Blair Valley.

GPS COORDINATES

UTM Zone (WGS 84) 11S
Easting 555765
Northing 3655345
Latitude N 33° 2' 7"
Longtitude W 116° 24' 10"

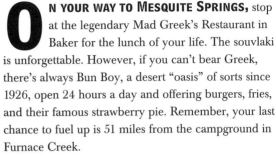

> *This campground is one of the few not overrun by large snowbird RVs in the winter.*

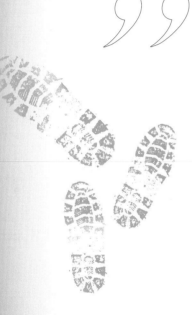

ON YOUR WAY TO MESQUITE SPRINGS, stop at the legendary Mad Greek's Restaurant in Baker for the lunch of your life. The souvlaki is unforgettable. However, if you can't bear Greek, there's always Bun Boy, a desert "oasis" of sorts since 1926, open 24 hours a day and offering burgers, fries, and their famous strawberry pie. Remember, your last chance to fuel up is 51 miles from the campground in Furnace Creek.

Despite its morbid name, Death Valley is a pretty lively place. For thousands of years Native Americans thrived on the shores of successive lakes that filled the basin. When the last lake dried up, the nomadic Shoshone camped in the valley near the springs in the winter and in the mountains in the heat of the summer. For the last thousand years, they lived on the ample game, mesquite beans, and pinyon nuts.

It took an overly eager forty-niner to dub the bountiful valley "Death Valley." He was one of a group of impatient argonauts who ignored their experienced wagon master and took a Native American trail in hopes of shaving miles off the trip. The group wound up bogged down in the sand around Furnace Creek. When rescued, the forty-niner theatrically exclaimed, "Good-bye, Death Valley!" as he turned his back on his own folly.

Seeing Death Valley for the first time is like seeing the earth without clothes. Immense land forms, volcanic craters, and rainbowed landscapes of salt flats and snowcapped mountains cover the area. There are original water springs, Ice Age fish, ghost towns, lost mines, plants found nowhere else in the world, and even a Spanish-Moorish castle, Scotty's Castle, built in the middle of nowhere.

Below Scotty's Castle lies the Mesquite Springs

RATINGS

Beauty: ✪ ✪ ✪ ✪ ✪
Privacy: ✪
Spaciousness: ✪ ✪ ✪ ✪
Quiet: ✪ ✪ ✪ ✪
Security: ✪ ✪ ✪ ✪ ✪
Cleanliness: ✪ ✪ ✪ ✪ ✪

Campground, set in the Grapevine Canyon wash. It has well-maintained tent and RV sites with fireplaces and tables. The campground offers flush toilets and spring-water spigots. You'll find soft, sandy spots to pitch your tent and a beautiful view of the entire valley with snow-covered Telescope Peak rising 11,000 feet in the south.

Far enough from Stovepipe Wells and the golf course at Furnace Creek, Mesquite Springs Campground is not heavily camped except during Easter holiday. Still, it's not a bad idea to phone the Ranger Station near the campground at (760) 786-3200 to check on availability. It's a hefty drive back to Furnace Creek and the Texas Spring campground, which is your alternative. Remember too, that the only supplies in Death Valley are sold in Furnace Creek and Stovepipe Wells.

A visit to Scotty's Castle is a half-day affair. After the guided tour, the bookstore, and a stroll around the grounds, find the tree-shaded picnic tables for lunch. Nearby are Ubehebe Crater and Little Hebe, which constitute another half-day excursion.

In Death Valley, distance shrinks. The locals think nothing of driving 60 miles for a cup of coffee. In that spirit, the ghost town of Rhyolite, and Beatty, with its gambling casinos (64 miles away), are just around the corner, as are the mining towns of Tonopah and Goldfield.

Hiking around Mesquite Springs Campground is fun. Because of the terrain, it's almost impossible to get lost. Still, always take a lot of water with you, even if you are just going out for a stroll. The last time we camped there it was a full moon, and we could see the entire valley far below us gleaming in the light. From the trees near the spring, an owl swooped down and rose again with a little creature in its claws.

This is a good campground for children. The campground roads are easily navigable and safe, so bring their bicycles. (Remember: Death Valley is long-haul driving country.) There is swimming at Stovepipe Walls. The fee is a nominal $2 per person.

KEY INFORMATION

ADDRESS:	Mesquite Springs Campground Death Valley National Park P.O. Box 579 Death Valley, CA 92328
OPERATED BY:	National Park Service
INFORMATION:	(760) 786-3200; www.nps.gov/deva
OPEN:	Year-round
SITES:	40
EACH SITE HAS:	Picnic tables, fireplaces
ASSIGNMENT:	First come, first served; no reservations
REGISTRATION:	At entrance
FACILITIES:	Water, flush toilets, sanitary disposal station
PARKING:	At individual sites
FEE:	$12, plus $20 7-day park pass
ELEVATION:	1,800 feet
RESTRICTIONS:	*Pets:* On leash only *Fires:* In fireplaces *Alcohol:* No restrictions *Vehicles:* RVs or trailers

MAP

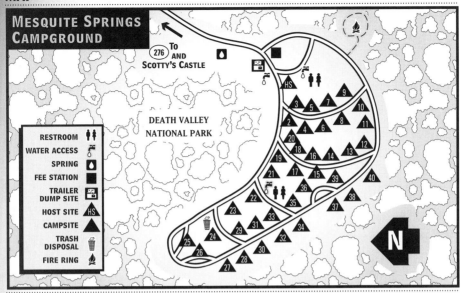

GETTING THERE

From L.A., drive 65 miles east on I-10 to I-15. Go north 135 miles to Baker. From Baker, drive 86 miles north on CA 127 through Shoshone to Death Valley Junction. From there drive 29 miles on CA 190 to Furnace Creek. Head north 51 miles to Mesquite Springs Campground on the left.

GPS COORDINATES

UTM Zone (WGS84) 11S
Easting 467187
Northing 4091065
Latitude N 36° 57' 54"
Longtitude W 117° 22' 07"

THE **E**AST **M**OJAVE **ISN'T HALF** as wild and woolly today as it was in 1826 when Jedediah Smith came through with a pack of angry Mojave Native Americans on his trail. Ambushed crossing the Colorado River, Smith lost half his trading party to Mojave war clubs before he forted up in a thicket of cottonwoods. With only five Kentucky rifles, Smith and his mountain men discouraged the Mojaves enough with pinpoint rifle fire to escape and run for their lives across the East Mojave Desert.

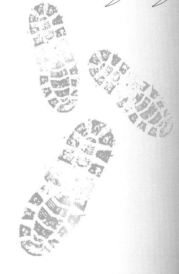

Come to Mid Hills Campground for the spring bloom. The back roads are good for mountain biking.

It was August 18 and hotter than Hades. Tormented by thirst, the men "found some relief from chewing slips of the Cabbage Pear," Smith wrote in his diary. Men dropped from exhaustion and could not go on until water could be found and brought back to them. "It seemed a more fitting abode for fiends than any living thing that belongs to our world," wrote James Ohio Pattie, another famous trapper of Smith's day. Traveling by night, the men spent the days by springs that Smith vaguely remembered from his trip the year before. They followed the Old Mojave Trail—a trading route used by the Mojave for hundreds of years—and passed close by present-day Mid Hills Campground on their terrified flight across the desert wastes toward the Cajon Pass.

Nowadays, Mid Hills Campground is about the most pleasant place to spend some time in these parts. Set in rolling country among juniper and pinyon pine, Mid Hills is high enough to get snow, sometimes in May. I liked Site 14 for its views of the mountains through the trees and the many places to pitch a tent. Also enticing are the sites situated on the edge of a drop, with a view of the vast Cima Dome and the Kelso Dunes to the south.

Between the Providence and New York mountains, Mid Hills is the trailhead for the 8-mile hike to Hole-in-the-Wall Campground. Start at Mid Hills for a

RATINGS

Beauty: ✿ ✿ ✿
Privacy: ✿ ✿ ✿ ✿ ✿
Spaciousness: ✿ ✿ ✿ ✿
Quiet: ✿ ✿ ✿ ✿ ✿
Security: ✿ ✿
Cleanliness: ✿ ✿ ✿

ADDRESS:	Mid Hills Campground Mojave National Preserve 222 East Main Street Suite 202 Barstow, CA 92311
OPERATED BY:	National Park Service
INFORMATION:	(760) 928-2572; www.nps.gov/moja
OPEN:	Year-round (forget summer, though)
SITES:	26
EACH SITE HAS:	Fire rings, picnic tables
ASSIGNMENT:	First come, first served; no reservations
REGISTRATION:	At entrance
FACILITIES:	Pit toilets, trash cans, water (usually)
PARKING:	At site
FEE:	$12
ELEVATION:	5,600 feet
RESTRICTIONS:	*Pets:* On leash only *Fires:* In fire rings *Alcohol:* No restrictions *Vehicles:* 2 per site (the unpaved road to the campground is unsuitable for RVs) *Other:* Bring firewood or charcoal.

mostly downhill trek and arrange a return ride. A mile or so into the hike, there is a small, cold-water seep coming from beneath a dead juniper. I can imagine Jedediah Smith and his boys lying around there in the blazing sun waiting for the Mojave to beset them.

The trail features incredible views, and the land changes quickly from the pine-juniper forest to desert—with bright, delicate desert flowers for a short while in springtime. At the end of the hike, coming up a blind canyon, there are rings set in the rock that help get you over the steep sections of the hike.

Hole-in-the-Wall Campground is the only organized alternative to Mid Hills. When both campgrounds are full, campers may tent in "previously disturbed areas." This option gives you a couple thousand attractive campsites from which to choose. In fact, just around the corner from Hole-in-the-Wall Campground, you'll find a whole series of turnoffs on the incredibly scenic Wild Horse Canyon Road. Be sure to drive it—you'll see cholla and wildflowers growing on volcanic slopes and rocky mesa, sage, and the pinyon-juniper woodland of Mid Hills Campground.

When visiting the Mojave National Preserve, water is your paramount concern. Count on at least a gallon per person, per day. Phone the park before you leave to see which campground has water. When we visited, Hole-in-the-Wall had water, but Mid Hills didn't.

Gasoline is also scarce. Fill up when you can. It is illegal to burn anything you find in the preserve—even dead wood—so bring your own wood or charcoal. Wind is another consideration. Mid Hills is protected by trees and hills, but Hole-in-the-Wall is out in the open. Bring earplugs if you can't sleep through the noise of a tent flapping in the breeze.

Between the Mitchell Caverns (tours available weekdays at 1:30 p.m., weekends at 10 a.m. and 3 p.m.), Kelso Dunes, Cinder Cones National Natural Landmark, Cima Dome, Fort Piute, Whiskey Pete's casino, hotel, restaurant, and truck stop just across the border in Nevada, and Bun Boy and the Mad Greek's Restaurant in Baker, you could easily spend a week around the Mojave National Preserve.

MAP

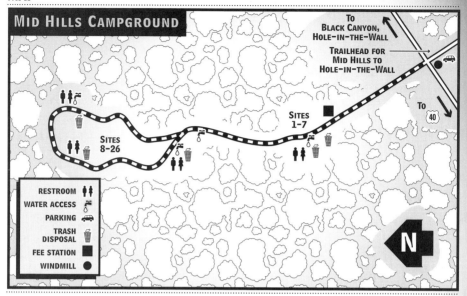

On the way to the Mojave National Preserve, stop at the California Welcome Center off I-15 (4 miles south of Barstow; [760] 253-4782) for maps, guidebooks, and information. Spring is the season to visit Mojave National Preserve. Not only are the riots of flowers in bloom, but also the desert is scoured clean by winter, leaving a crust over the sand to keep down the dust.

GETTING THERE

From L.A., take I-10 east to I-15 north to I-40. Go east on I-40 near Essex, then take the Essex Road exit and drive 10 miles north to Black Canyon Road. Then drive 9 miles north, following the signs to the campground.

GPS COORDINATES

UTM Zone (WGS 84) 11S

Easting 646474

Northing 3879053

Latitude N 35° 2' 37"

Longtitude W 115° 23' 39"

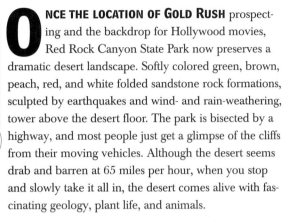

*Explore the Mojave
Desert from Ricardo
Campground,
where Joshua trees
stand sentry.*

ONCE THE LOCATION OF GOLD RUSH prospecting and the backdrop for Hollywood movies, Red Rock Canyon State Park now preserves a dramatic desert landscape. Softly colored green, brown, peach, red, and white folded sandstone rock formations, sculpted by earthquakes and wind- and rain-weathering, tower above the desert floor. The park is bisected by a highway, and most people just get a glimpse of the cliffs from their moving vehicles. Although the desert seems drab and barren at 65 miles per hour, when you stop and slowly take it all in, the desert comes alive with fascinating geology, plant life, and animals.

In the desert, there is little privacy between campsites, but at Red Rock, Joshua trees, creosote shrubs, a variety of cacti, and the sandstone formations do provide some landscape buffering. Many sites are spaced a comfortable distance apart, while others are clustered more tightly together. If you don't mind hauling your stuff to your campsite, check out Site 7, an easy 300-foot walk from the parking area. We snagged this spot, and were rewarded with the most private desert campsite we've ever seen. The desert sand is coarse here, and it feels great to walk around barefoot, but be cautious for scorpions and rattlesnakes.

The Mojave Desert is like an oven from late spring to autumn, and early spring is the favored season. When we visited in late April, there were still good displays of lingering wildflowers prominent on the bare, sandy desert floor near our campsite, including sand verbena, fiddlenecks, and golden gilia.

Serious star watchers camp here—park staff post sky charts on the campground information boards, and we saw folks with massive scopes, setting up around dusk. The campground's bowl-shaped orientation, tilted slighty uphill from the Ranger Station, allows good views of the sky, particularly to the north.

RATINGS

Beauty: ✿ ✿ ✿ ✿
Privacy: ✿ ✿
Spaciousness: ✿ ✿ ✿
Quiet: ✿ ✿ ✿
Security: ✿ ✿ ✿
Cleanliness: ✿ ✿ ✿ ✿

When you're exploring the desert, a good routine is to start your day early, hike when the temperatures are still cool, then return to camp for some serious afternoon lollygagging. Red Rock's easiest hikes are brief tours through the area, accompanied by interpretive guide pamphlets available at most trailheads. Introduce yourself to the area by exploring the visitor center exhibits at the Ranger Station, then walking the very short Ricardo Nature Trail, which begins across the parking lot from the Ranger Station. Stretch your legs more on Desert View Nature Trail, at the edge of the campground, or Hagen Canyon Trail, which starts from a trailhead right off the highway. To get to the other trailheads on the east side of the highway, you'll need to drive a short distance. Red Cliffs Nature Trail requires only about 30 minutes to complete, and is a good place to admire the park's namesake iron oxide–stained cliffs, and some of the area's best wildflowers in early spring. Another popular hike, indicated on the park map as "scenic cliffs," is closed from February to May to protect nesting birds; ask at the visitor center about this route's status.

In the afternoon when the sun is high in the sky and the temperatures soar, you'll want to find some shade, so keep that in mind as you scope the campground for your site. On a hot afternoon we escaped to the shade of a small cluster of Joshua trees and tried to read, but were constantly distracted by birds. Wrens, finches, larks, flycatchers, and warblers are all frequently spotted in the park, along with two omnipresent desert birds, ravens and vultures. At night and early in the morning we heard an owl hooting nearby.

Once you exhaust the park's series of short hikes, there's not much else to do in the immediate area, so unless you're committed to total relaxation in a desert environment, you'll likely find a two- or three-night stay just right. If you want to go for a drive, head south and east of California City to the Desert Tortoise Natural Area, a Bureau of Land Management–run preserve where you can look for tortoises on a 2-mile hike. Be sure to pick up all the food you need at Mojave. Stater Brothers grocery store on CA 14 is the last chance for

ADDRESS:	Red Rock Canyon State Park PO Box 26 Cantil, CA 93519 Mojave Desert State Park 43779 15th Street West Lancaster, CA 93534
OPERATED BY:	California State Parks
INFORMATION:	(661) 942-0662; www.parks.ca.gov
OPEN:	Year-round, but too hot in summer
SITES:	50 sites for tents and RVs up to 30 feet
EACH SITE HAS:	Fire ring, picnic table
ASSIGNMENT:	First come, first served; no reservations
REGISTRATION:	At Ranger Station
FACILITIES:	Pit toilets, drinking water, firewood for sale, 2 wheelchair-accessible sites
PARKING:	At individual sites
FEE:	$12
ELEVATION:	2,600 feet
RESTRICTIONS:	*Pets:* On leash, in campground only, not allowed on trails *Fires:* In established pits/rings only *Alcohol:* No restrictions

MAP

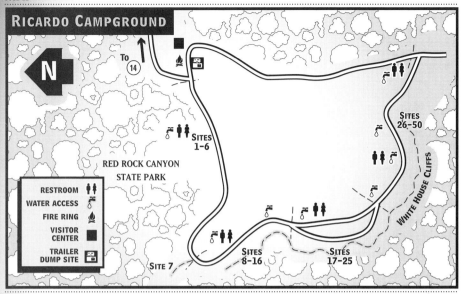

RICARDO CAMPGROUND

N

To (14)

SITES 1-6

RED ROCK CANYON
STATE PARK

SITES 26-50

WHITE HOUSE CLIFFS

RESTROOM
WATER ACCESS
FIRE RING
VISITOR CENTER
TRAILER DUMP SITE

SITE 7

SITES 8-16

SITES 17-25

GETTING THERE

From the town of Mojave in Kern County, drive north on CA 14 for 24 miles, then turn left into the park, following the sign for Ricardo Campground. Continue another 2 miles to the Ranger Station and campground.

anything substantial, but you can pick up ice at the small store in Jawbone, a few miles south of the park. A Bureau of Land Management off-road vehicle area sprawls on the west of Red Rock, and from some sites you can occasionally hear the hum of dirt bikes. Some off-road enthusiasts set up base camp at Red Rock, but we found the jeep and dirt bike noise no more intrusive than that of the lumbering RVs and massive pickup trucks that are common to campgrounds these days.

GPS COORDINATES

UTM Zone (WGS84) 11S
Easting 409807
Northing 3914708
Latitude N 35° 22' 18"
Longtitude W 117° 59' 34"

19
SADDLEBACK **BUTTE** **STATE** PARK CAMPGROUND

SADDLEBACK **B**UTTE **S**TATE **P**ARK is little known, well run, and very convenient to the Los Angeles area. It lies just over the hill on the Antelope Freeway, an oasis in the creeping suburbia of Antelope Valley. I like the park because of its proximity to Los Angeles. It's perfect for a quick desert-camping trip if you don't have time to drive to Joshua Tree National Park or Anza-Borrego Desert State Park.

The San Gabriel Mountains to the south block out the L.A. smog. You'll see wildflowers among the park's many Joshua trees from February through May. In fact, the park was once called Joshua Tree State Park, but everyone confused it with Joshua Tree National Park, so they renamed it after Saddleback Butte, a mountain a few hundred yards to the east of the campground.

Look for horned larks and alligator lizards, as well as the golden eagle, desert tortoise, and the usual compendium of desert creatures. Examine the Joshua tree, which John C. Fremont dubbed the "most repulsive tree in the vegetable kingdom" in 1844. Later, J. Smeaton Chase likened the poor tree to "a misshapen pirate with belt, boots, hands, and teeth stuck full of daggers . . ." Lighten up a bit, dudes. I think the *Yucca brevifolia,* as the Joshua tree is known botanically, is as beautiful as can be and as strong as it has to be to survive in a harsh environment.

The Joshua tree is a natural supermarket. Woodrats gnaw off the lower leaves to make nests. Weevils lay eggs in the tree's terminal bud, which causes the multiple branching effect. Yucca moths are the plants' sole pollinator, and in turn, lay their eggs in the flower. Butcher birds (the loggerhead shrike) hang their prey out to dry on the sharp leaves, and woodpeckers dig holes in the limbs looking for insects. In the past, Native Americans ate the flowers, raw or roasted, and then ate the seed pods. They made sandals and

> *This is a fine first desert trip for children from Los Angeles.*

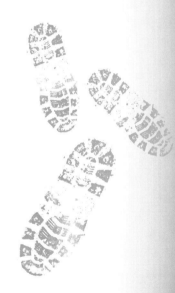

RATINGS

Beauty: ☆ ☆ ☆
Privacy: ☆ ☆ ☆
Spaciousness: ☆ ☆ ☆
Quiet: ☆ ☆
Security: ☆ ☆ ☆ ☆ ☆
Cleanliness: ☆ ☆ ☆ ☆

ADDRESS: Saddleback Butte
State Park
17102 East Avenue J
Lancaster, CA 93535

OPERATED BY: California State
Parks

INFORMATION: (661) 942-0662;
www.parks.ca.gov

OPEN: Year-round

SITES: 50; 1 reserved for
groups

EACH SITE HAS: Barbecue grill,
picnic table, shade
screens, fire rings

ASSIGNMENT: First come, first
served; no reserva-
tions for individual
sites; group site is
reservable

REGISTRATION: By entrance; reserve
by phone, (800)
444-6777, or online,
www.reserve
america.com.

FACILITIES: Water, flush toilets,
dump station

PARKING: At site

FEE: $12

ELEVATION: 2,700 feet

RESTRICTIONS: *Pets:* On leash only,
in campground only
Fires: In established
pits/rings only
Alcohol: No
restrictions
Vehicles: $5 for extra
vehicle; RVs and
trailers up to 30
feet; no hookups

carrying nets from the fiber in the leaves, and the roots were used to make dyes and medicines. In all, the Joshua tree is a useful plant. It's most attractive in spring, covered with and surrounded by flowers, or in winter, when the sunlight hits its tufted branches covered with snow.

The area around Saddleback Butte State Park was once antelope country. Imagine the Piute Native Americans on top of the 3,600-foot butte scouting for herds of pronghorn antelope on the distant horizon. Then came the iron horse, the railroad, in the 1870s. Not only were there hordes of trigger-happy sportsmen on the train blazing away at anything that moved, but the pronghorn antelope also had their own fatal flaw: for some reason, they couldn't cross railroad tracks. Something in the pronghorn make-up wouldn't let them. So, unable to follow their normal grazing patterns, many starved to death.

The pronghorn are among the fastest animals in the world. Three feet high at the shoulder, the pronghorn can run 65 miles per hour in short bursts and 35 miles per hour for 4 miles. There are a few left in sagebrush country on the Modoc Plateau, but it's an uphill fight.

The trail up Saddleback Butte starts in the campground and moves due east up an easy grade, passing through creosote and Joshua trees. It winds around the alluvial fan and climbs up the saddle-shaped hunk of granite. From the top, you can see the other buttes in the area. All of them, including Saddleback Butte, are the tops of granite mountains silted up by the alluvial plain, which is Antelope Valley. To the north is Edwards Air Force Base, and farther west are Lancaster and the Antelope Valley California Poppy Reserve, where poppies blanket entire hillsides in brilliant orange. This area is worth a visit. Remember to phone ahead at (661) 724-1180 to find out when the poppies are in bloom. From the Antelope Valley Freeway in Lancaster, take the Avenue I exit and drive 15 miles west to the reserve.

The Antelope Valley Indian Museum is also worth a stop. It is a folk museum of various Native American tribes and houses a unique southwestern collection. It is

MAP

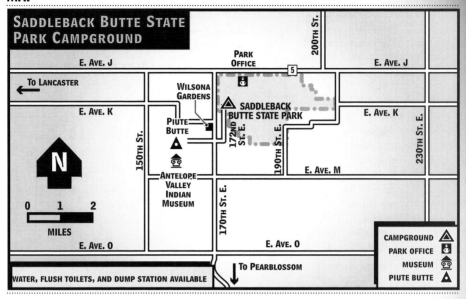

open weekends from 11 a.m. to 4 p.m., mid-September to mid-June. To get to the museum, take 170th Street 3 miles south from the Park to Avenue M. Go west for 1 mile to the museum sign. You won't regret it.

Saddleback Butte State Park is first come, first served; however, the park is only really busy one or two weekends during peak flower time in the spring. Don't camp here in the summer. October and November are pleasant times to visit. Check the weather report and wind conditions before you leave; it can really blow here. In anticipation, there are windscreens by every campsite.

GETTING THERE

From L.A., drive north on I-5 to I-14 north to Lancaster. Turn east on Avenue J (County Highway N5) and drive 17 miles to the park entrance.

GPS COORDINATES

UTM Zone (WGS 84) 11S

Easting 424423

Northing 3837512

Latitude N 34° 40' 36"

Longtitude W 117° 49' 30"

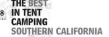

20
VALLECITO
REGIONAL PARK
CAMPGROUND

Vallecito Regional Park is good for children, winter camping, and Old West lore.

NATIVE **AMERICANS LIVED** on the site of Vallecito Regional Park for thousands of years. Then came the Spanish conquistadors, Kit Carson and General Kearny, the forty-niners and the Conestoga wagons, and then, the stagecoaches. Vallecito oasis is on the main southern route westward from St. Louis, which goes through Texas to avoid mountains and bad weather. The last water is near Yuma on the Colorado River, and then there's nothing but a hundred miles of trackless, dry wasteland.

One anonymous forty-niner quoted on a park billboard describes Vallecito this way:

> *Imagine the weary traveler, ragged and dirty, surrounded by barren, burning sands, with no green thing upon which to rest his eye. See him toiling to ascend the sandy rise. He reaches the top and in the distance he sees the green countenance of Vallecito. Gratitude to God fills his heart when he reaches the spot where he can lie down in green pastures and refresh himself.*

Ripping through the desert in an air-conditioned car, you won't get quite the same sensation, but Vallecito is truly a magical spot. Surrounded by mountains of heat-blasted rock, Vallecito is soft, green, and filled with wildlife. Behind the campground is a privately owned preserve, a mesquite forest alive with bees and birds.

The campground is simple. Under the trees, near the restored stage station and cemetery on the only high ground, sit the 22 tent-only spots—well away from the RV and trailer area. The restrooms are simple and clean. The ranger is on top of everything. This is a beautiful, well-run camp! It is a perfect place to come with children for a first-time camping trip or to frame nights spent camping in Anza-Borrego Desert State Park primitive campsites.

RATINGS

Beauty: ☆ ☆ ☆
Privacy: ☆ ☆
Spaciousness: ☆ ☆ ☆
Quiet: ☆ ☆ ☆
Security: ☆ ☆ ☆ ☆ ☆
Cleanliness: ☆ ☆ ☆ ☆ ☆

There is a playground for little ones. You can spot rabbits hopping through the campground, as well as road runners, lizards, and quail. Bring binoculars and a bird book. To cook up a meal, tote charcoal and grillables. If you forget, you can buy supplies at the two stores nearby—Butterfield Ranch and Agua Caliente. Both places also have swimming pools available for a small fee.

The reconstructed stage station is fascinating and full of history involving hauntings, lost gold, and murder. One man rode his white horse into the station one night and shot his brother dead at the bar. Another story tells of a young woman who came off the stagecoach and expired in the station. An elaborate wedding dress was found in her baggage. She was buried in it, and sometimes her apparition is seen wafting through the rooms of the stage station at dusk. Some days, hundreds of Conestoga wagons camped around the station as the oxen and settlers gathered strength for the final push over the mountains.

The stagecoaches ran 24 hours a day. At night a man on horseback rode ahead carrying a lantern to light the way. A six-horse team pulled the stage. There were quick stops to change horses and only one meal per day for the passengers. The 2,800-mile trip from St. Louis to San Francisco took 24 days. Imagine more than 100 miles per day in a stagecoach with no springs! No wonder people alit in San Francisco battered and bruised and swore never to ride another stage.

The two times I've slept in the park, the place was deserted. However, the ranger warned me that on Easter or other big weekends the park fills up. Most sites are first come, first served, so plan to arrive early. The rest of the time, Vallecito is a welcome drop-in relief from the other organized campgrounds in the area, such as Borrego Palm Canyon and Tamarisk Grove.

Nearby hiking is available. You can bushwhack in the desert across the road or trek up the sandy wash of Smuggler Canyon. A short car ride away, you'll find Emigrant Trail and Blair Valley to the north, and trailheads at Bow Willow in the south. A good gem-hunting trip is located south, on S-2 almost to Ocotillo. On the

KEY INFORMATION

ADDRESS:	Vallecito Regional Park Department of Parks and Recreation 5201 Ruffin Road Suite P San Diego, CA 92123-1699
OPERATED BY:	County of San Diego
INFORMATION:	(858) 694-3900, www.sdparks.org
OPEN:	June–September
SITES:	22 for RVs, trailers, and tents; 22 for tents only
EACH SITE HAS:	Picnic table, barbecue, fireplace
ASSIGNMENT:	www.co.sandiego.ca .us/parks/
REGISTRATION:	By entrance
FACILITIES:	Water, flush toilets, playground
PARKING:	At individual sites
FEE:	$15
ELEVATION:	1,500 feet
RESTRICTIONS:	*Pets:* On 6-foot leash; must be attended at all times; $1 fee *Fires:* In established barbecue stoves or fire rings *Vehicles:* RVs or trailers *Alcohol:* Beer and wine; nothing over 40 proof *Other:* No generators

MAP

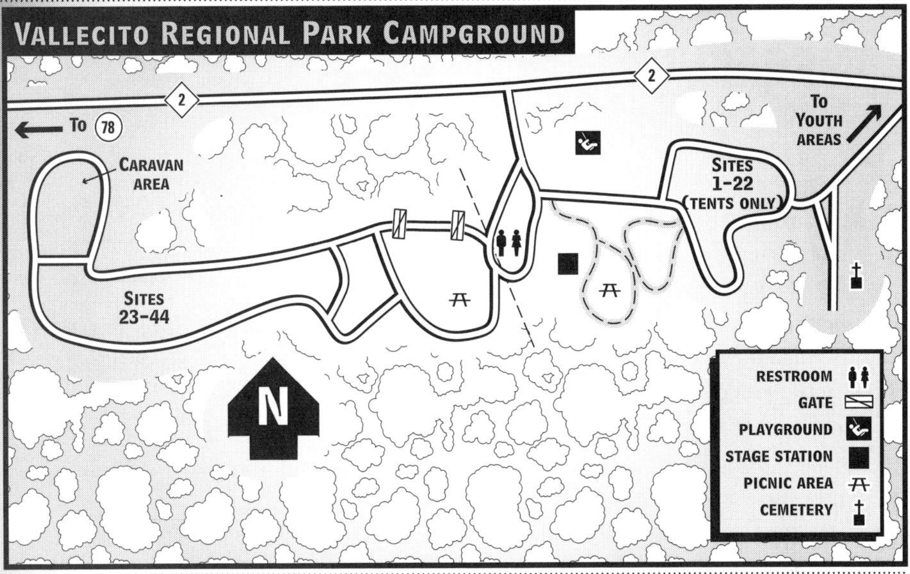

VALLECITO REGIONAL PARK CAMPGROUND
2
2
To 78
To
YOUTH
AREAS
CARAVAN
AREA
SITES
1-22
(TENTS ONLY)
SITES
23-44
N
RESTROOM
GATE
PLAYGROUND
STAGE STATION
PICNIC AREA
CEMETERY

GETTING THERE

From L.A., take I-10 east to I-15. Go south to Temecula. Take CA 79 east to Julian and CA 78 down Banner Grade to Scissors Crossing. Then take S-2 about 18 miles to the park.

left is Shell Canyon Road. Drive as far as you can, then hike. The canyon is filled with fossil shells and onyx. Go east on S-80 4 miles past Ocotillo and turn left on Painted Gorge Road. Again, be careful of the sand. There are agate and jasper immediately on the left and fossils in the hills to the right farther up the mountain. This is a good hike even if you aren't interested in gems.

GPS COORDINATES

UTM Zone (WGS 84) 11S
Easting 560713
Northing 3648727
Latitude N 32° 58' 31"
Longtitude W 116° 21' 1"

21
WHITE TANK CAMPGROUND

WHY IS THE ARBORESCENT tree yucca (*Yucca brevifolia*) called the Joshua tree? I have it on good authority that a group of Mormons was laboring across the trackless wastes, under a blazing sun, when they entered a *Yucca brevifolia* forest. Out of nowhere a cloud blocked the sun. In their ecstasy, the pioneers proclaimed the strange plants Joshua trees, referencing the Old Testament prophet who called on God block the sun. Indeed, the tufted branches resemble an old, robed prophet imploring the heavens with raised hands.

I visited Joshua Tree National Park with a group of friends. We taxed our bones trekking up the strenuous trail to the top of Ryan Mountain. When my wife, who stopped speaking to me on the rigorous ascent, saw the snows on Mount San Jacinto and the Little San Bernardinos and the Lost Horse Valley spread below, she relented graciously and acknowledged that the carrot was worth the climb.

Then came White Tank Campground, where we found a cozy campsite in an alcove in the rocks. The pitch was soft and sandy, and boulders blocked the wind. We packed a lunch basket and set out to find White Tank using the following instructions:

"Take the Arch Rock Trail. When you come to the sign that designates 'Arch,' stop and look around. To the south, 20 feet away, see the slabs of sandwiched rock. Climb over those keeping the Arch Rock on the left, and you'll come down into sandy sheltered White Tank, a prime place for a picnic."

Indeed we did, and with minimal difficulty. We learned to slide down the steep rocks on our bottoms. The quartz monzonite boulders found here stick tight to blue jeans and sneakers, simplifying an otherwise hairy climb.

> *White Tank has incredibly beautiful winter and spring camping, but don't get caught here in the summer!*

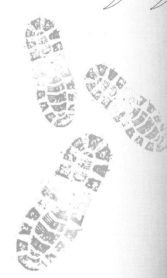

RATINGS

Beauty: ☆ ☆ ☆ ☆ ☆
Privacy: ☆ ☆ ☆
Spaciousness: ☆ ☆ ☆
Quiet: ☆ ☆ ☆ ☆
Security: ☆ ☆ ☆ ☆
Cleanliness: ☆ ☆ ☆ ☆

KEY INFORMATION

ADDRESS:	White Tank Campground Joshua Tree National Park 74485 National Park Drive Twentynine Palms, CA 92277
OPERATED BY:	National Park Service
INFORMATION:	(760) 367-5500, www.nps.gov/jotr
OPEN:	Year-round
SITES:	15
EACH SITE HAS:	Picnic table, fire ring
ASSIGNMENT:	First come, first served; no reservations
REGISTRATION:	At entrance
FACILITIES:	Pit toilets, bring plenty of water
PARKING:	At site
FEE:	$10; $15 to enter Joshua Tree National Park
ELEVATION:	3,800 feet
RESTRICTIONS:	*Pets:* On leash only *Fires:* In fireplaces (bring your own firewood or charcoal) *Alcohol:* No restrictions *Vehicles:* RVs up to 27 feet *Other:* All vegetation in park protected; limit of 6 people, 2 tents, and 2 vehicles per site; no water provided.

White Tank lived up to its billing. It was warm in the sun and cool under the huge rocks, and the sand was as white and clean as a Bahama beach. What a lunch!

Afterward, we backtracked to the "Arch" sign. Somewhere out there was Grand Tank, a body of water with colonies of fairy and tadpole shrimp. How did they get here? The friendly ranger at the Park Headquarters in Twentynine Palms told me their ancestors hitched a ride to Grand Tank on the feet of migrating ducks!

To find Grand Tank, head downhill from the "Arch" sign and follow the trail that goes across a wash and up a hill. After a bit, the trail splits. We went left. "Follow the strong trail!" I urged my companions, who suggested I engrave that on my tombstone when we reached a dead end. Backing up, we climbed west to find the "strong trail" again. We saw birds diving into what we discovered were Grand Tank and the stream running south from it.

Vindicated at last, I identified white-winged doves and house finches circling the water. Grand Tank is about 15 feet deep. I looked in vain for the much-vaunted, hitchhiking shrimp. As the day went on, I led my group of doubting Thomases south along the stream and safely back to camp.

That night there was a full moon. With field glasses we examined the figure on the lunar surface to see if it was indeed a long-eared rabbit as the Chinese believe or, in fact, the man widely publicized in my youth. Swayed perhaps because the next day was Easter, I conceded that it might be a rabbit after all.

A mile-and-a-half back toward the Park Headquarters in Twentynine Palms is Belle Campground, just as charming as White Tank and as accessible to the California Riding and Hiking Trail. The trail, which crosses Cottonwood Springs Road between the two campgrounds, is best in early morning and evening, when twilight gives the flat desert rich hues and texture. Along with Ryan Campground in Lost Horse Valley, Belle and White Tank offer the best camping in Joshua Tree. Other campgrounds are overrun by RVs and rock climbers in fall and spring—the only times you want to be caught alive in this desert.

MAP

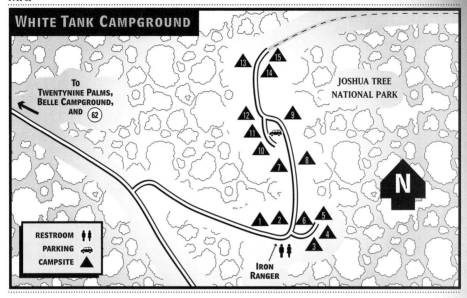

WHITE TANK CAMPGROUND

To
TWENTYNINE PALMS,
BELLE CAMPGROUND,
AND (62)

JOSHUA TREE
NATIONAL PARK

N

RESTROOM
PARKING
CAMPSITE

IRON
RANGER

It's not a bad idea to check the weather report before you come to Joshua Tree. The Santa Ana winds come in the fall, and winds come from the coast in the winter, bringing rain. When it really blows, you must decide whether to tie your tent to the car or actually get into the car. Sometimes it will blow for hours—sometimes days.

In any season, you can dine at the wonderfully idiosyncratic Twentynine Palms Inn adjacent to the Park Headquarters on the Oasis of Mara, Twentynine Palms' original raison d'être. Walk around and look at the ducks on the pond, the truck garden fenced by palm fronds, and guest cabins that once belonged to miners.

GETTING THERE

From L.A., take I-10 east to CA 62 past Banning over the San Gorgonio Pass. Go north and east to Twentynine Palms. Drive 8 miles south on the Utah Trail to the intersection with Cotton-wood Springs Road. Then go left (south) 1.5 miles to the campground.

GPS COORDINATES

UTM Zone (WGS 84) 11S
Easting 590831
Northing 3761006
Latitude N 33° 29' 9"
Longtitude W 116° 1' 0"

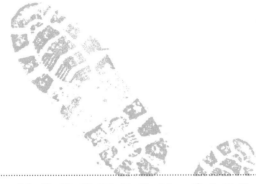
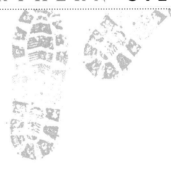

THE NORTHERN SIERRAS

DRIVE THROUGH TORRID VISALIA on any July afternoon and you'll know why the Yokut and Monache Native Americans fought over the summer camps by Atwell Mills, where it is pleasant during the day and cool at night. They built little, round thatched houses and carpeted the floor with oak leaves and ferns. The women gathered most of the food, and the men spent most of their time in the sweat house. Summer was a time of plenty for them, with pine nuts, fish, manzanita cider, wild tobacco, and an occasional deer. The deer were stalked by one man alone, wearing a deer disguise and using arrows poisoned with rattlesnake venom. The Native Americans here led a great life, but it went like the wind when the white man appeared on the scene, hot after the riches of Mineral King.

The road up to Atwell Mill follows the old Native American trail. It's steep, but near Atwell Mill the ground levels out. This is one of the few areas around flat enough to camp and work on. A. J. Atwell of Visalia thought so, and built a small sawmill in the meadow below the campground. You can still see the remains of the mill's steam engine near the stumps of the giant sequoias it helped reduce to shingles, grape stakes, and fence posts.

Steam engines tore their way through the American West. Anywhere there was fuel for the boiler, the engine could do the work of hundreds of men. Some Native Americans thought engines were a breed of devil, and, for them, I think that was true.

Folks knew how to build a steam engine for a thousand years before they could make iron durable enough for steam boilers. Finally, in England in 1600, a blacksmith experimented with burning coke in order to make a better frying pan and discovered the process

> *This is one of the two best backcountry campgrounds in Sequoia National Park.*

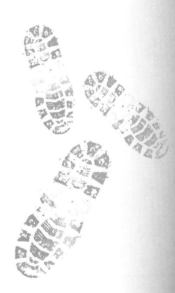

RATINGS

Beauty: ✿ ✿ ✿ ✿ ✿
Privacy: ✿ ✿ ✿ ✿ ✿
Spaciousness: ✿ ✿ ✿ ✿ ✿
Quiet: ✿ ✿ ✿ ✿
Security: ✿ ✿ ✿ ✿ ✿
Cleanliness: ✿ ✿ ✿ ✿ ✿

ADDRESS:	Atwell Mill Campground Sequoia and Kings Canyon National Parks 47050 Generals Highway Three Rivers, CA 93271-9700
OPERATED BY:	National Park Service
INFORMATION:	(559) 565-3341; www.nps.gov/seki
OPEN:	Memorial Day– October 31 (weather permitting)
SITES:	21
EACH SITE HAS:	Picnic table, fire pits, bear boxes
ASSIGNMENT:	First come, first served; no reservations
REGISTRATION:	At entrance
FACILITIES:	Water, pit toilets, wheelchair-accessible sites
PARKING:	At site
FEE:	$12 camping fee, $20 for 7-day park entrance fee
ELEVATION:	6,650 feet
RESTRICTIONS:	*Pets:* On leash only, not allowed on trails *Fires:* Allowed in fireplaces; may be prohibited when fire danger is high *Alcohol:* No restrictions *Vehicles:* 1 vehicle per site; 6 people maximum per site; no RVs or trailers *Other:* Don't leave food out, use bear boxes; 14-day stay limit.

that produces high-grade iron. That discovery ultimately enabled deforestation at Atwell Mill.

Still, there's a magic to Atwell Mill. It's in the scarred stumps more than a hundred years old. It's in the young sequoias reaching up in the shade of cedars, pines, and white firs. This is classic mountain camping.

All winter, the campsites are cleansed by 20 feet of snow. In the summer, the air smells clean and rich with the odor of redwood and pine. Walk up the little ridge above the campground and watch the sun set on the mountains across the Kaweah River. Or better yet, head down the Atwell Hockett Trail between campsites 16 and 17. The trail passes the supine steam engine on the right and heads over the hill. About 100 yards from the metal sign banning firearms and dogs, go to the right, about 30 yards down, to the famous Native American bathtubs. The rock outcropping there is a great place to have lunch or a sundowner. There, manzanita open up the forest to give you a great view of the mountains and sky.

Back on the main trail, carry on past little Deadwood Creek to East Fork Kaweah River gorge with its giant sequoias and mist kicked up by the falls. Rough trails head up either side of the gorge for more private picnicking and sunning spots. Or, keep walking the many miles up to Hockett Meadows.

Another good hike is up the Atwell Redwood Trail. From the campground, walk back down the Mineral King Road you drove up on and find the trailhead at a curve about 500 yards down. Hike up the mountain into the Atwell Grove sequoias. Three of these trees are gigantic. At their feet are the bracken fern that the Native Americans used to carpet the floors of their houses. Keep hiking up and to the left along the ridge to Paradise Peak. The hike is about 9 miles round-trip and should take you all day.

Remember, when you leave Three Rivers you are bidding adieu to ice-and-beer country. So, ice up. Remember, block ice lasts about three days to cube ice's one day.

The sign where the Mineral King Road takes off from CA 198 should tell you if Atwell Mills and Cold

MAP

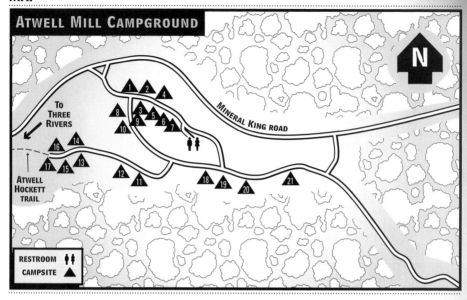

ATWELL MILL CAMPGROUND

N

To THREE RIVERS

MINERAL KING ROAD

ATWELL HOCKETT TRAIL

RESTROOM

CAMPSITE

Springs have campsites available. However, this sign is not always up to date, so phone the Ranger Station in Mineral King at (559) 565-3341 to make sure. It is a three-hour round-trip, so you don't want to arrive and not find a campsite. On the Mineral King Road turn your lights on. It helps traffic see you a split second earlier, which means a lot on this hairy road. Bring bug repellent in August to deter biting pests. And remember to use the bear boxes!

GETTING THERE

From L.A., take I-5 north over the Tejon Pass to CA 99. Drive north on CA 99 past Bakersfield. Take CA 65 north to Exeter. Go east (right) on CA 198 to Three Rivers. Go 3 miles and turn right on the Mineral King Road. It's about 20 miles to Atwell Mill. Plan on the trip taking 1.5 hours.

GPS COORDINATES

UTM Zone (WGS84) 11S
Easting 350550
Northing 4036712
Latitude N 36° 27' 51"
Longtitude W 118° 40' 05"

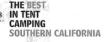

23
BUCKEYE CAMPGROUND

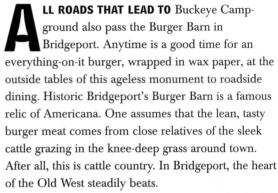

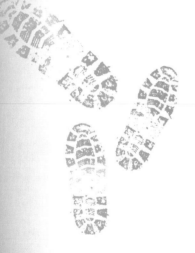

"Come for fishing, hiking, the magnificent rocky slopes, and far-off glaciers."

ALL ROADS THAT LEAD TO Buckeye Campground also pass the Burger Barn in Bridgeport. Anytime is a good time for an everything-on-it burger, wrapped in wax paper, at the outside tables of this ageless monument to roadside dining. Historic Bridgeport's Burger Barn is a famous relic of Americana. One assumes that the lean, tasty burger meat comes from close relatives of the sleek cattle grazing in the knee-deep grass around town. After all, this is cattle country. In Bridgeport, the heart of the Old West steadily beats.

There are four loops to the campground. The first loop you come to on the left, sites 42 through 68, has the campground host (employed by L & L Inc. concessionaires). Bundles of wood are sold at the host station. You continue up the hill for the other three loops. Two have pit toilets, and the other has flush toilets but was closed the last time I was up there.

At 7,000 feet, Buckeye is Big Country camping. The air smells of pine, dust, and cold, rushing water. Buckeye Creek runs right past the campground. The mountain wildflowers grow from the sandy needled floor among the sage. You look up and see the rocky slopes and, farther on, the white of the glaciers on the peaks: it's cowboy country. A horse trail cuts right by the camp. The sites are mostly unoccupied; the pitches are scoured clean by the winter. This is an excellent place to camp.

Fishing is not bad on Buckeye Creek between the two bridges—that's where the fish are stocked. You can hike on over to Twin Lakes and rent a boat. Go for the big brown trout. In 1987 somebody caught the state record, a 26.8 pounder, here. However, most of the folks I saw with fish had caught little rainbows. The water-skiing on Upper Twin scares away some of the trout, so the best fishing is on Lower Twin. I talked with

RATINGS

Beauty: ✪ ✪ ✪ ✪ ✪
Privacy: ✪ ✪ ✪ ✪ ✪
Spaciousness: ✪ ✪ ✪ ✪ ✪
Quiet: ✪ ✪ ✪ ✪ ✪
Security: ✪ ✪ ✪ ✪ ✪
Cleanliness: ✪ ✪ ✪ ✪ ✪

one old-timer who said the best time to come for the browns is in May, when it is cold and windy. Troll with rapelas (three- to four-inch minnow), he advised. I threw in some salmon eggs and didn't get a nibble.

Another big draw at Buckeye Campground is the hot springs. They are by the stream down from the campground. It's best to get in your car and drive down the hill. Take your first left and climb a slight hill. There is a slanting parking area immediately on the right. Climb down the steep slope to the hot pools by the river below. This can be fun. Wear shoes with some bite since the footing is slippery. Sometimes the pools are empty, sometimes filled with fun-loving folks. Last time I was there, one pool was occupied by a lone, naked, whalelike chap who looked to me boiled-lobster pink. I chose to wear bathing apparel. I sat first in the hot pool, then sat in Buckeye Creek to cool off.

Good hiking can be had right out of camp. Buckeye Campground is in a V between the two branches of Buckeye Creek. The two hikes follow the two branches upstream and ultimately swing around and join one another, so you can make up to a 16-mile loop. Bring fishing gear since there are elusive brown trout and rainbow in the upper reaches; use local worms and try the pools behind beaver dams. The trailhead to the two hikes is up above the campground loops. Just walk up the access road (newly tarred and graveled) and it will dead-end into a horse corral and the trailhead (see the map posted there).

One trail heads west along the right-hand branch of Buckeye Creek. This trail follows an erstwhile wagon road through flowered meadows and pine forest. The trail up the left-hand branch of Buckeye Creek can be accessed from the campground's left-hand loops (looking west). Just walk to the creek and head up the fisherman's trail. Otherwise, walk from the trailhead a few hundred yards until the trail winds left up a ridge to the stream. The wildflowers in July were all over the place—lupine, shooting star, paintbrush. Watch the campground notice board for ranger wildflower nature walks—they are fun.

Bring ice—the nearest supplies are at Doc and Al's,

KEY INFORMATION

ADDRESS: Buckeye Campground Humboldt–Toiyabe National Forest Bridgeport Ranger Station HCR 1 Box 1000 Bridgeport, CA 93517-0595

OPERATED BY: U.S. Forest Service

INFORMATION: (775) 331-6444; www .fs.fed.us/r4/htnf

OPEN: May–October (depending on road and weather conditions)

SITES: 65 sites

EACH SITE HAS: Picnic table, fire ring

ASSIGNMENT: First come, first served; no reservations

REGISTRATION: At entrance to each loop

FACILITIES: Flush and vault toilets, drinking water

PARKING: At individual site

FEE: $11

ELEVATION: 7,500 feet

RESTRICTIONS: *Pets:* On leash only *Fires:* In fire ring *Alcohol:* No restrictions *Vehicles:* RVs up to 30 feet *Other:* Don't leave food out

MAP

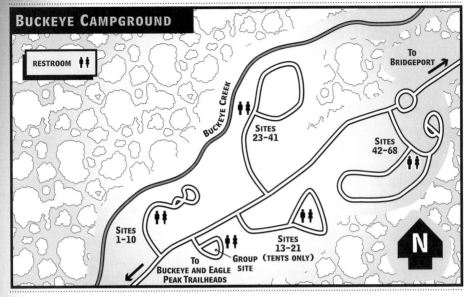

BUCKEYE CAMPGROUND

RESTROOM

BUCKEYE CREEK

SITES 23–41

To BRIDGEPORT

SITES 42–68

SITES 1–10

To BUCKEYE AND EAGLE PEAK TRAILHEADS

GROUP SITE

SITES 13–21

(TENTS ONLY)

N

GETTING THERE

From Bridgeport, take the Twin Lakes Road southwest to Buckeye Road on the right by Doc and Al's Resort. Go 4 miles on the dirt road to the campground.

GPS COORDINATES

UTM Zone (WGS84) 11S
Easting 294579
Northing 4234766
Latitude N 38° 14' 22"
Longtitude W 119° 20' 53"

or Bridgeport. Think about cooling your beer and sodas in the stream. Or buy a cheap Styrofoam cooler, fill it with ice, duct-tape it shut, and put it in a cool place. Mind the bears. Put all your foodstuff in the car trunk when you go off. Bears are busy tending their cubs and looking for chow during camping season. By fall, bears max out, eating 20,000 calories every day in preparation for hibernation.

Good side trips from Buckeye are to Bodie (bring food and water), Mono Lake, and the Virginia Creek Settlement (once part of Dogtown, a gold-rush mining camp) for a look around and a meal. Go gem hunting near Bridgeport. Head 3.3 miles north from Bridgeport on CA 182, and turn right on Forest Service Road 046. Head out exploring (avoid any active mines) for quartz crystals, chalcopyrite, and pyrite.

24
COLD SPRINGS CAMPGROUND

COLD **S**PRINGS **C**AMPGROUND is the most beautiful campground in Southern California. Down by the gorgeous Kaweah River, this campground is situated in the shadows of Sawtooth and Mineral Peaks, Needham and Rainbow Mountains, and to the south, Miners Ridge. Winter scours out the valley so it feels brand new every summer. A waterfall cuts through the walk-in camping area. The rush of the water is white noise; you'll sleep like a baby. I love this campground.

Back in the 1870s, miners took one look at the rocks in Mineral King and rushed in. What excited them was the contact zone between reddish metamorphics and grayish granite. So sure of silver was Thomas Fowler, a wealthy rancher from Tulare County, that he bet his entire fortune on his Empire Mine, boasting that he would pay off America's national debt and then buy Ireland to free it from the tyrannical British. First, Fowler built the road into Mineral King. A local reporter described the mine's opening: "I doubt that General Grant felt more proud when he rode into Richmond than did honest Tom Fowler when he rode into Mineral King. . . ."

Of course, the mine went bust. Avalanches swept away the mine, the town, and the mile-long bucket tramway to the stamp mill in the valley. All that was left of Fowler's dream was the road, and folks used it to get away from the brutal heat in the Central Valley below. In 1893, the federal government declared the area part of the Sierra Forest Preserve.

In the 1960s, the Forest Service considered building a major ski resort at Mineral King. The Walt Disney Corporation proposed a resort with a skiing capacity of 10,000 persons daily. Widespread opposition and lawsuits from environmental groups ensued,

> *The most beautiful campground in the adjacent Sequoia and Kings Canyon National Parks.*

RATINGS

Beauty: ✿ ✿ ✿ ✿ ✿
Privacy: ✿ ✿ ✿ ✿ ✿
Spaciousness: ✿ ✿ ✿ ✿ ✿
Quiet: ✿ ✿ ✿ ✿ ✿
Security: ✿ ✿ ✿ ✿ ✿
Cleanliness: ✿ ✿ ✿ ✿ ✿

ADDRESS: Cold Springs
Campground
Sequoia and Kings
Canyon National
Parks
47050 Generals
Highway
Three Rivers, CA
93271-9700

OPERATED BY: National Park
Service

INFORMATION: (559) 565-3341,
www.nps.gov/seki

OPEN: Memorial Day–late
October (weather
permitting)

SITES: 40

EACH SITE HAS: Picnic table,
fire pit, bear box

ASSIGNMENT: First come, first
served; no
reservations

REGISTRATION: At entrance

FACILITIES: Water, pit toilets,
coin-operated
showers, wheelchair-
accessible sites

PARKING: At site

FEE: $20 for 7-day park-
entrance fee

ELEVATION: 7,500 feet

RESTRICTIONS: *Pets:* On leash only,
not allowed on trails
Fires: Allowed in fire
pits; fires may be
restricted during
high fire season
Alcohol: No
restrictions
Vehicles: No RVs or
trailers
Other: No harming
marmots; keep food
in bear boxes, not in
tents or cars; 14-day
stay limit.

and finally, in 1978, Congress made Mineral King part of Sequoia National Park.

Now Mineral King is famous for its marmots. These little devils have a penchant for gnawing on auto parts from early spring to about mid-July. They chew on hoses, fan belts, and electrical wiring. Some people bring chicken wire to put around their cars. Unless you park on a hard surface and seal the edges of the wire with piled rocks, so the marmots can't dig their way in, the chicken wire just makes a big marmot playpen. In springtime, leave your car in the hikers' parking lot in Atwell Mill Campground, and get a lift up to Mineral King. As the summer progresses, the chewing ends, and marmot-safe parking reaches higher altitudes until it is safe to park at the trailheads in Mineral King. It's a good idea to phone the rangers and ask about the latest on marmot activity. You don't want to pay $250 to get towed to Three Rivers.

Don't hate the humble marmot. It's a brave little rodent. With hair standing on end and long claws at the ready, the feisty marmot clatters his sharp teeth and whistles loudly at enemies. Marmots are superbly created to survive in a harsh environment. Their bodies afford "clear and cogent arguments of the wisdom and design of the Author" (Robert Boyle, 1688). And, it's against federal law to use poison or other substances to kill, deter, or otherwise foil marmots from car-gnawing.

Remember to get supplies in Three Rivers. Put drinks in a gunnysack and store them in the Kaweah River. That'll chill the cans.

Think about using the walk-in campsites at Cold Springs, nestled in a corner between the Kaweah River and a waterfall that pours down to the river. To access the walk-ins, take the second right loop and follow it to the parking lot at the end. Bring rucksacks to carry your stuff the hundred yards or so into the sites. There is piped water and a pit toilet in among the sites.

A trail (3 miles round-trip) heading east from Cold Springs Campground (trailhead between sites 6 and 7) directs you along a signed nature trail. I found out that corn lilies are also called skunk cabbage and that

MAP

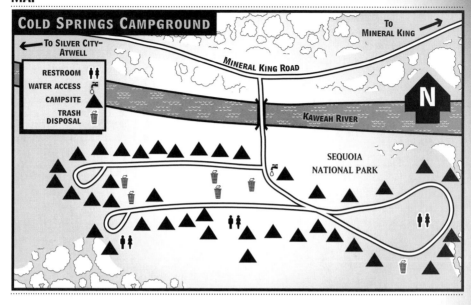

COLD SPRINGS CAMPGROUND

To Silver City–Atwell

To Mineral King

Mineral King Road

Kaweah River

RESTROOM

WATER ACCESS

CAMPSITE

TRASH DISPOSAL

SEQUOIA NATIONAL PARK

N

juniper seeds need to be partially digested by birds in order to sprout, which means they grow far away from their parent trees. Stay on the trail, which hits a road to the right of Mineral King Village and arrives at the trailhead for Tufa Falls (another easy hike) and other destinations heading up Farewell Canyon.

Plan on spending more than a day or so in Mineral King. You could spend most of the summer hiking out of Cold Springs Campground, but give yourself a day or two to get used to the altitude.

GETTING THERE

From L.A., take I-5 north over the Tejon Pass to CA 99. Take CA 65 north to Exeter. Go east (right) on CA 198 to Three Rivers. Three miles past Three Rivers turn right onto Mineral King Road. It's about 25 miles to Cold Springs Campground. Plan on the 25-mile trip taking 1.5 hours.

GPS COORDINATES

UTM Zone (WGS84) 11S

Easting 355585

Northing 4035222

Latitude N 36° 27' 05"

Longtitude W 118° 36' 41"

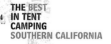

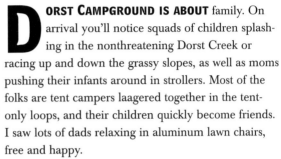

> *This is a good summer family campground with wonderful side trips.*

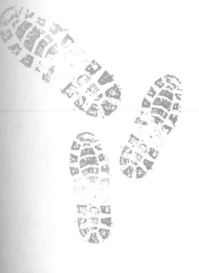

DORST **CAMPGROUND IS ABOUT** family. On arrival you'll notice squads of children splashing in the nonthreatening Dorst Creek or racing up and down the grassy slopes, as well as moms pushing their infants around in strollers. Most of the folks are tent campers laagered together in the tent-only loops, and their children quickly become friends. I saw lots of dads relaxing in aluminum lawn chairs, free and happy.

On the Generals Highway, Dorst is a perfect base camp from which to explore Giant Forest, Grant Grove, and, farther afield, Cedar Grove. Not too far away is Hume Lake with big-time swimming prospects. A quick run will get you groceries or grits at Lodgepole or Stony Creek Lodge.

An early explorer of what is now Sequoia National Park, William Brewer, wrote: "Such a landscape! A hundred peaks in sight over thirteen thousand feet—many very sharp, deep canyons, cliffs in every direction almost rivaling Yosemite, sharp ridges almost inaccessible to man, on which human foot has never trod—all combined to produce a view the subliminity of which is rarely equal, one which few are privileged to behold."

The Park Service has fought hard to keep it that way. In fact, one of their biggest fights was against sheep. The mountains were perfect for sheepherding. The sheep ran amok through the forests, eating everything in sight, ripping it all up by the roots. Kings Canyon was fast becoming a high-altitude desert. The park superintendent called out the U.S. Cavalry, and still the sheep and shepherds kept coming. Only when the superintendent hit on the strategy of banning sheep on one side of the Sierras and shepherds on the other side was the ovine feeding frenzy discouraged.

A great hike from Dorst Campground leads to the Muir Grove of giant sequoias. Even if you poke along,

RATINGS

Beauty: ✿ ✿ ✿ ✿
Privacy: ✿ ✿ ✿
Spaciousness: ✿ ✿ ✿ ✿
Quiet: ✿ ✿ ✿ ✿
Security: ✿ ✿ ✿ ✿
Cleanliness: ✿ ✿ ✿ ✿ ✿

the round-trip shouldn't take more than four hours. Find the trailhead at the Dorst Campground amphitheater (follow the beehive symbol west). The trail is signed and leads you up through white firs and sugar pines, then over a ridge to the Muir Grove giants. The good news is that the return trip is mostly downhill.

Another nearby hike is up Little Baldy. The trailhead is 1.6 miles south of the Dorst Campground entrance on Generals Highway. Park in the pull-off area at the Little Baldy Saddle and head northeast. Two hard miles later you're on the bare granite Little Baldy summit. It's not a great place to be in a thunderstorm, but it's fine for lying in the noon sun.

If you tire of Dorst Campground family fun, or if you arrive and the campground is full, an alternative lies in the neighboring Sierra National Forest. Leave Dorst Campground and turn left up Generals Highway toward Grant Grove. Turn right on Big Meadow Road and drive about 5 miles to Big Meadows Campground Number 3. Pass up the heavily used Big Meadows Campground Numbers 1 and 2. Below Number 3, Boulder Creek spills down rocky chutes and gathers in pools. There is good dipping there, but be careful. The rock is slippery.

Or, pick up a fire permit as you pass the Hume Lake Forest Service Station on CA 180, and you can camp in one of literally thousands of wonderful, potential sites for hunkering down overnight.

Farther down the white-knuckle Big Meadow Road is Horse Corral Meadow, where, in 1922, a cowpoke named Jessie Agnew killed the last grizzly bear in California, claiming it was after his cattle. Imagine, killing the last California grizzly, our state animal!

Back at Big Meadows Campground, look for a brown, fiberglass post marking a trailhead. From here, you can hike up to Weaver Lake or Jennie Lake. Take the trail about 2 miles to Fox Meadow where there's a small wooden sign and a trail register. Weaver Lake is straight ahead about 1.5 miles. The trail to Jennie Lake, to the right, heads south 5 miles.

The best way into Dorst Campground is up CA 180 from Fresno. The other road in, through Three

KEY INFORMATION

ADDRESS: Dorst Campground Sequoia and Kings Canyon National Parks 47050 Generals Highway Three Rivers, CA 93271-9700

OPERATED BY: National Park Service

INFORMATION: (559) 565-3341, www.nps.gov/seki

OPEN: June–September (depending on road and snow conditions)

SITES: 218

EACH SITE HAS: Picnic table, fire pits, bear boxes

ASSIGNMENT: Site-specific reservations accepted; reservations recommended

REGISTRATION: At entrance; reserve by phone, (800) 365-2267, or online, www.recreation.gov.

FACILITIES: Water, flush toilets, wheelchair-accessible sites

PARKING: At site

FEE: $20, plus $1.50 reservation fee

ELEVATION: 6,700 feet

RESTRICTIONS: *Pets:* On leash only
Fires: In fire pits; fires may be prohibited during high fire danger
Alcohol: No restrictions
Vehicles: 1 per site; maximum 6 people per site
Other: Keep food in bear boxes, not in tents or cars; 14-day stay limit.

MAP

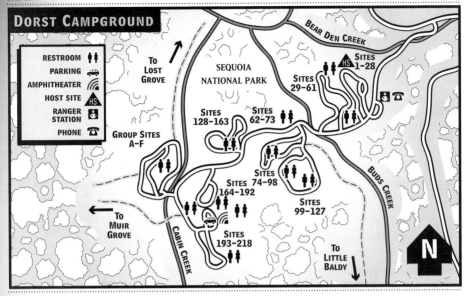

DORST CAMPGROUND

RESTROOM	👫
PARKING	🚗
AMPHITHEATER	📡
HOST SITE	HS
RANGER STATION	🔧
PHONE	☎

To LOST GROVE

SEQUOIA NATIONAL PARK

BEAR DEN CREEK

SITES 1–28

HS

SITES 29–61

SITES 128–163

SITES 62–73

GROUP SITES A–F

SITES 74–98

SITES 164–192

BUDS CREEK

SITES 99–127

To MUIR GROVE

CABIN CREEK

SITES 193–218

To LITTLE BALDY

N

GETTING THERE

From L.A., take I-5 north over the Tejon Pass to CA 99. Drive north on CA 99 to Fresno. Turn right on CA 198 and drive to Kings Canyon National Park. Turn right (south) on Generals Highway and drive 16 miles to Dorst Campground on the right.

Rivers, is a bear. It's narrow, slow, and scary. When you arrive at Dorst Campground, check out all the loops. I camped in a loop allowing trailers and found the campsite much roomier and more private than the sites on the tent-only loops.

Try to camp at Dorst long enough to relax and get to know the area. I think three days is a minimum. One day just doesn't get it. Camping has its own clock, and it runs slowly.

GPS COORDINATES

UTM Zone (WGS84) 11S
Easting 338059
Northing 4056031
Latitude N 36° 38' 10"
Longtitude W 118 ° 48' 41"

DRIVING FROM **LOS ANGELES** to East Fork, you'll go through Mojave, the desert, and then the Owens Valley, a graben, according to geologists, which means it's a 100-mile-long, 5-mile-wide trench between the Sierras on the west and the White-Inyo Mountains on the east. It's a magical place, and the Native Americans coined the name Inyo, meaning "dwelling place of the great spirit."

It is a land of dramatic contrast and incredible beauty, where mountain and desert meld into breathtaking scenery, and glaciered peaks tower over shimmering alkali flats. Tumbling mountain streams become lost in the desert, and gem-like lakes shimmer against deep pine forests.

East Fork Campground on Rock Creek lies right in the heart of the beast. Rock Creek is in a glacial cirque (basin) and drops 6,000 feet and 20 miles to the Owens River. On the way to East Fork, you'll pass Bishop (the last good town for shopping); don't forget to stop at Mahogany Smoked Meats on US 395 as you leave town. Buy some smoked pork chops for that night's dinner. Gnaw on some world-famous slab jerky as you drive up the infamous Sherwin Grade (or Vaporlock Grade as the old-timers called it). You'll climb 24 miles and about 3,000 feet to Tom's Place, where you will turn south on Rock Creek Road.

Stop at Tom's Place. It's a restaurant/store/bar/cabin complex where you can get fishing information and the bait the trout are hitting that day. You can buy last-minute camping supplies or eat some of the gut-plug pancakes for breakfast or gravy-soaked chicken fried steak for dinner.

Head up Rock Creek Road. Pass French Camp Campground. It's a lovely campground by the creek. It's almost 1,500 feet lower than East Fork Campground, which makes it a good place to camp in the

> *Some say East Fork features the best camping in the Sierras.*

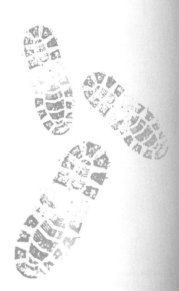

RATINGS

Beauty: ✿ ✿ ✿ ✿ ✿
Privacy: ✿ ✿ ✿ ✿ ✿
Spaciousness: ✿ ✿ ✿
Quiet: ✿ ✿ ✿
Security: ✿ ✿ ✿ ✿ ✿
Cleanliness: ✿ ✿ ✿ ✿ ✿

KEY INFORMATION

ADDRESS:	East Fork Campground Inyo National Forest 351 Pacu Lane Suite 200 Bishop, CA 93514
OPERATED BY:	U.S. Forest Service
INFORMATION:	(760) 873-2400; www .fs.fed.us/r5/inyo/
OPEN:	May–November
SITES:	133
EACH SITE HAS:	Picnic table, Fireplace, food-storage cabinet
ASSIGNMENT:	Some sites require reservations; others are first come, first served.
REGISTRATION:	At entrance; reserve by phone, (877) 444-6777, or online, www .reserveusa.com.
FACILITIES:	Water, pit toilets
PARKING:	At site
FEE:	$18, plus $1.50 reservation fee
ELEVATION:	9,000 feet
RESTRICTIONS:	*Pets:* Allowed *Fires:* In fireplace *Alcohol:* No restrictions *Vehicles:* RVs up to 22 feet *Other:* 14-day stay limit

spring, when the flowers are out down below and East Fork is still socked in with winter cold. At East Fork Campground the bloom arrives later in the summer.

As Owens Valley writer Mary Austin observed, "Well up from the valley, at the confluence of canyons, are delectable summer meadows. Fireweed flames about them against gray boulders; streams are open, go smoothly about the glacier slips, and make deep bluish pools for trout. Pines raise statelier shafts and give themselves room to grow gentians, shinleaf, and little grass of Parnassus in their golden checkered shadows; the meadow is white with violets, and all outdoors keeps the clock."

Find the entrance to East Fork Campground at about 9,000 feet (auto parts stores often sell car altimeters for less than $20, which are surprisingly accurate and fun to watch). The campground is down on Rock Creek. Most of the sites on the creek are lovely, but in the open, and have RV-size parking spots. Other sites, back up from the creek, are small and private. The parking spots are half a dozen yards from the campsites, which are mostly private and secluded in little copses of pine, brush, and aspen.

When I was there in late September, the aspen leaves were turning gold. When the wind blew they shimmered so prettily in the sunlight and made a soft, tinny clatter as they shook. The creek was well stocked. Happy fishermen tromped back to their campfires with strings of nice-sized trout for dinner. At night, the cold snapped, and, in the morning, our camping neighbors all exclaimed how nippy it was.

The hardy ridges above the riparian campground are covered with isolated foxtail pines. The creek goes north and south, so the sun is quick to set at night and slow to rise in the morning. At 9,000 feet, you really want the sun and will walk with your morning coffee to find it. A nice evening walk is across the bridges to the other side of the creek. Go to Site 108, the host's site, and across the access road you'll find the first bridge. There is fine fishing here.

A solid hike is up the creek to Rock Creek Lake. The trail leaves on the north side of the campground by Site 82 and goes all the way to Rock Creek Lake,

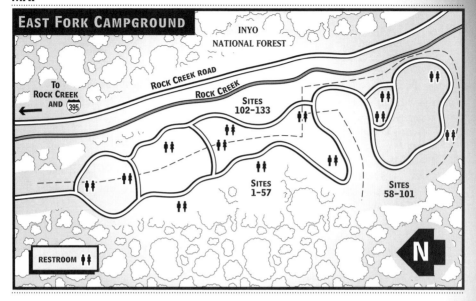

EAST FORK CAMPGROUND

INYO
NATIONAL FOREST

ROCK CREEK ROAD

ROCK CREEK

To
ROCK CREEK
AND (395)

SITES
102-133

SITES
1-57

SITES
58-101

RESTROOM

N

passing some small campgrounds and a resort before
hitting the lake and trailheads to the high country.

Above Rock Creek Lake, you'll find Mosquito
Flat. You can drive there and park at 10,250 feet. From
there, it's an easy day hike into the John Muir Wilderness and Little Lakes Valley. The valley is a pretty
glacial trough below 13,000-foot peaks. Bring your
wildflower book because the meadows up there are
loaded with wildflowers.

GETTING THERE

From L.A., take I-5 north to
CA 14. Go north to US 395
near Inyokern. Continue
north on US 395 to Bishop.
From Bishop, drive 24 miles
north on US 395 and exit to
the west at Tom's Place onto
Rock Creek Road. Drive
5 miles up Rock Creek Road
to the campground.

GPS COORDINATES

UTM Zone (WGS84) 13S
Easting 348059
Northing 4149908
Latitude N 37° 29' 01"
Longtitude W 118° 43' 07"

27
FAIRVIEW
CAMPGROUND

Fairview Campground offers the best tent camping in the Lake Isabella area.

ABOUT 60,000 YEARS AGO, a glacier flowing down an earthquake slip fault cut the U-shaped Upper Kern Canyon. Look southward along the Upper Kern Canyon and you can see how the glacier carved out the canyon, giving it rounded shoulders. In the Lower Kern Canyon, below Lake Isabella where the glacier didn't flow, the shoulders of the canyon are sharp and V-shaped.

Fairview Campground, near the head of the Upper Kern Valley, is the best camping spot in the area. It's set down by the river, well below the road and any traffic noise, with the mountains towering around. The sites are so well planned it's hard to decide where to camp. The last time I was there it was spring, and the snow level was down to 5,000 feet, but it was warm and sunny down in the campground.

All the flowers were out—most ostentatiously the purple yerba santa. We made a tea out of its leaves, which the Native Americans thought was good for coughs, colds, asthma, and the like. Pretty bitter stuff. I've also heard that the leaves, when pounded into a poultice, cure sores. The Spanish used the leaves as tobacco, for chewing and smoking. Others claim that you can chew the leaves to quench thirst. After the first bitter taste subsides, you'll feel a sweet, cooling sensation. I tried it, and it wasn't too bad.

By our campsite, we found a flowering flannel bush (*Fremontia californica*) with brazen yellow flowers bright against the white water of the Kern. All night, the strong current rattled the rocks on the river bottom. In the morning, the ranger, who came by to collect our $15, admired our flannel bush and reported that the bark can be brewed and gargled to relieve a sore throat.

Fairview has always been blessed. The Native Americans used it as a fall and spring campground. In

RATINGS

Beauty: ✿ ✿ ✿ ✿ ✿
Privacy: ✿ ✿ ✿ ✿
Spaciousness: ✿ ✿ ✿ ✿
Quiet: ✿ ✿ ✿ ✿
Security: ✿ ✿ ✿ ✿
Cleanliness: ✿ ✿ ✿ ✿

the late 1800s, Stony Rhymes and Lucien Barbeau had a cow camp on the bend of the river. In 1910, Matt and Lupie Burlando moved to Fairview and built the Fairview Lodge. They rented rooms to tourists who came for fishing and hunting. Matt built a swinging bridge (you can still see it today) across the river to the natural hot springs on the west side and ran packing trips into the backcountry. After Matt and Lupie's children reached school age, the entire family moved down to Kernville to be near the school. Fairview went back to being a cow camp for a while before Johnny McNally opened McNally's Steakhouse. Johnny was an amazing rodeo rider and a deputy sheriff, and his wife, Pauline, could shoot a running buck with a rifle from the back of a galloping horse.

To reach McNally's from the campground, walk south along the river 50 yards. You'll find McNally's Steakhouse, the hamburger hut, and the gas station/grocery store. We loaded up on beer, hot dogs, and ice at the store and then hunkered down at the outside picnic tables for some rousing chili burgers before heading across the suspension bridge on a diet-redeeming hike along Flynn Trail. (See the map and handout sheet on the display by the parking lot near the hamburger stand.) You'll find access here for the Tobias Trail as well. Maybe the best short day hikes here are on the Whiskey Flat Trail, which runs from the bridge down to the north end of Burlando Road in Kernville. The trail parallels the west side of the river and runs through high chaparral, digger pines, and oak. There are wonderful places along the trail for picnicking. Put down a blanket and snooze while the river runs below you. I've heard there's good fishing here. Another good hike is up the trail to Salmon Creek Falls. The marked trailhead is a mile or so south of Fairview to the east.

One word of warning about the Kern River: it is very dangerous. When I was last there in May, it was running way above its natural banks. Camping there with children is only advisable if they are sternly warned and constantly watched. The water is cold, and the current is strong. If you're camping with children, go down below on Lake Isabella. I especially

ADDRESS:	Fairview Campground Sequoia National Forest c/o California Land Management P.O. Box 1640 Kernville, CA 93238
OPERATED BY:	U.S. Forest Service
INFORMATION:	(559) 784-1500; www.fs.fed.us/r5/sequoia
OPEN:	April–November
SITES:	55
EACH SITE HAS:	Fire ring, picnic table
ASSIGNMENT:	First come, first served; reservations recommended
REGISTRATION:	Host collects on rounds; reserve by phone (at least 3 days in advance), (877) 444-6777, or online, www.recreation.gov.
FACILITIES:	Water, vault toilets, wheelchair-accessible sites
PARKING:	At site
FEE:	$17–$19, plus $1.50 reservation fee
ELEVATION:	3,500 feet
RESTRICTIONS:	*Pets:* On leash only *Fires:* In fireplaces *Alcohol:* No restrictions *Vehicles:* RVs up to 45 feet

MAP

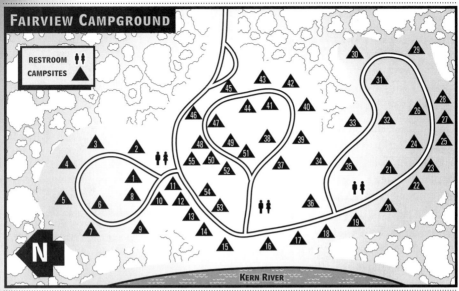

FAIRVIEW CAMPGROUND

RESTROOM
CAMPSITES

KERN RIVER

N

GETTING THERE

From L.A., take I-5 north to CA 99 past Bakersfield. Take CA 178 east to Lake Isabella. Take CA 155 north to Wofford Heights. Bear right to Kernville. From Kernville, drive north 16 miles on Kern River Highway–Sierra Road to Fairview Campground on the left.

recommend Tillie Creek Campground, which is pretty, safe, and flat. Bring the children's bicycles. There is even a playground. In the spring, good fishing can be found in the lake as well.

GPS COORDINATES

UTM Zone (WGS84) 11S
Easting 365437
Northing 3977090
Latitude N 35° 55' 44"
Longtitude W 118° 29' 30"

28
FOUR JEFFREY AND SABRINA CAMPGROUNDS

THE PRINCESS OF CAMPGROUNDS on Bishop Creek above Bishop is tiny Sabrina Campground perched on the lip of Lake Sabrina. At 9,000 feet, the view of the picture-perfect lake, the glaciered mountain peaks marbled with rusty red metamorphic rock, and the deep blue sky is breathtaking. Sit on the sunny patio of the Lake Sabrina Boat Landing and eat an incredible old-fashioned hamburger grilled up by the pleasant hostess. That's how you know you're not in Switzerland after all, but in the Wild West.

You'll see lanky anglers swigging Budweiser, a big husky dog asleep atop an up-turned aluminum boat, and cowpokes in ten-gallon hats stepping out of canoes, holding up six-pound trout, just caught, their bright colors catching the sun. Then, oddly, a pack train of laden llamas will file up the trail across the lake. Llamas? In the Wild West? Yes, apparently some of the local pack outfits use llamas. Indigenous to Peruvian high country, the llamas take to the Sierras like ducks to water.

Drive the vertiginous, short dirt road up to North Lake and check out North Lake Campground at the trailhead. No trailers, no RVs, only tents, but like Sabrina Campground and most of the campgrounds in the Bishop Creek area, it has few sites. The only campground around that has enough space to be a destination campground is Four Jeffrey, which is down the road from Sabrina Lake and to the right, on the spur road to South Lake.

Four Jeffrey is an impressive campground. The surrounding mountains are spare and dry, and the view is incredible, although not eye-poppingly stunning like the views from Sabrina and North Lake. The South Fork of Bishop Creek runs through the campground. Many of the sites are down by the water, which is alive with trout. Others are up the hill in low

> *Four Jeffrey Campground is the best destination campground in the Bishop Creek Drainage area.*

RATINGS

Beauty: ✪ ✪ ✪ ✪
Privacy: ✪ ✪ ✪ ✪
Spaciousness: ✪ ✪ ✪ ✪ ✪
Quiet: ✪ ✪ ✪ ✪ ✪
Security: ✪ ✪ ✪ ✪ ✪
Cleanliness: ✪ ✪ ✪ ✪ ✪

ADDRESS: Four Jeffrey and Sabrina Campgrounds Inyo National Forest 351 Pacu Lane Suite 200 Bishop, CA 93514

OPERATED BY: U.S. Forest Service

INFORMATION: (760) 873-2400; www .fs.fed.us/r5/inyo

OPEN: Four Jeffrey, April 26–October 29; Sabrina, May 15–October 15

SITES: Four Jeffrey 106; Sabrina 20

EACH SITE HAS: Picnic tables, fireplace

ASSIGNMENT: First come, first served; no reservations

REGISTRATION: At entrance; reservations by phone 4 days in advance (Four Jeffrey)

FACILITIES: Water, flush toilets, wheelchair-accessible sites

PARKING: At site

FEE: $19, plus $1.50 reservation fee

ELEVATION: 8,100 feet

RESTRICTIONS: *Pets:* On leash only *Fires:* In fireplace *Alcohol:* No restrictions *Vehicles:* RVs up to 22 feet *Other:* Four Jeffrey, 14-day stay limit; Sabrina, 7-day stay limit

brush. This area makes for good spring and early-summer camping. By fall, the hillside is muted and austere. I like that look, but others want the green of the pines.

Make Four Jeffrey the first-night destination campground in the Bishop Creek area. Chances of getting a site there are very good (the camping season at Four Jeffrey is two months longer than at Sabrina Campground). The next day, cruise around. Hit Sabrina Campground first, then North Lake Campground, then the other little campgrounds up and down the forks of Bishop Creek, and see if you find something you like better.

It was at Four Jeffrey Campground that I thrilled to the efficacy of the miner's lights sold in the camping stores. Ranging from cheap to pretty expensive, these babies are cinched around your head, so the light is on your forehead and the beam follows your eyes. My wife lost her contact lens somewhere around camp, and I went scouting for it. The light was better than ten camp lanterns. I found the lost lens with ease. Buy one of these lights. The more expensive ones are more comfortable, but the batteries and bulbs may be more difficult to purchase.

Part of my attraction to Four Jeffrey Campground has to do with survival. All the other campgrounds except little North Lake are by the streambed. And, the Bishop area is earthquake country. At 2:30 a.m. in March of 1872, a monster quake hit the Owens Valley. It was felt as far east as Salt Lake City, as far north as Canada, and as far south as Mexico. It shook old John Muir over in Yosemite Valley. He described the incident: "I was awakened by a tremendous earthquake, and though I had never enjoyed a storm of this sort, the strange thrilling motion could not be mistaken, and I ran out of cabin, both glad and frightened, shouting, 'A noble earthquake! A noble earthquake!' feeling sure I was going to learn something."

John Muir used to strap himself in the tops of pine trees during thunderstorms. He was lucky. Well, the 27 folks down in Lone Pine who died in the 1872 quake weren't so lucky. I figure a quake like that could happen again, and the dams up on Sabrina and

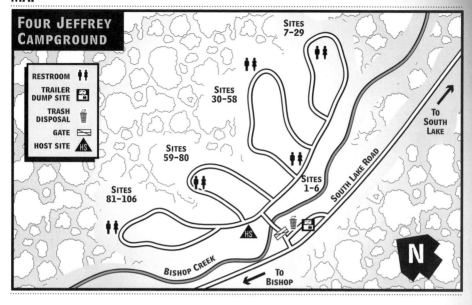

FOUR JEFFREY CAMPGROUND

RESTROOM	
TRAILER DUMP SITE	
TRASH DISPOSAL	
GATE	
HOST SITE	HS

SITES 7–29

SITES 30–58

SITES 59–80

SITES 81–106

SITES 1–6

SOUTH LAKE ROAD

TO SOUTH LAKE

BISHOP CREEK

TO BISHOP

N

South Lake would go pretty easily. I want to be sleeping on the high ground at Four Jeffrey Campground, so I can snooze right through the flood.

The best shopping is down the road in Bishop. The road in and out is good and fast. Bishop (named for Samuel A. Bishop, one of the area's original cattle ranchers) is a cow town recently encased in an ugly, fat pocket of fast-food franchises. Fortunately, Schat's Dutch Bakery is there for sheepherder bread. Jack's Waffle Shop is open for breakfast with locals and cowpokes; the Firehouse Grill still attracts tourists; and the Meadow Farms Country Smokehouse (north on US 395) still sells mahogany-smoked slab jerky, sweet 'n' hot jerky, cheddar jerky, and other varieties, so you can gnaw your merry way through the High Sierras!

GETTING THERE

From L.A., take I-5 north to CA 14 to US 395 near Inyokern. Continue north on US 395 for 123 miles to Bishop. Drive 13 miles south on CA 168 to South Lake Road. Go left for a mile or so to Four Jeffrey Campground. Sabrina Campground is another 4 miles south on CA 168 from that turnoff.

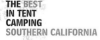

MAP

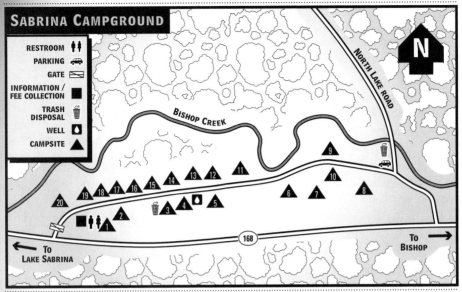

SABRINA CAMPGROUND

RESTROOM
PARKING
GATE
INFORMATION /
FEE COLLECTION
TRASH
DISPOSAL
WELL
CAMPSITE

BISHOP CREEK

NORTH LAKE ROAD

N

168

To
LAKE SABRINA

To
BISHOP

GPS COORDINATES

UTM Zone (WGS84) 11S

Easting 360705

Northing 4123628

Latitude N 37° 14' 56"

Longtitude W 118 ° 34' 14"

HORSE MEADOW CAMPGROUND is my favorite campground. I don't even know why. Maybe it's the long grind up the mountains, or the terrain, that dry, big-sky country look with the pines, boulders, and open, green meadows. Maybe I watched too many westerns when I was a child. The sky at Horse Meadow Campground just seems a little bit bluer.

The campsites at Horse Meadow are roomy and offer a great view. Salmon Creek runs through the campground and gurgles just enough to lull you to sleep. Below the meadow, it gathers in pools deep enough for you to take a freezing dip. When you hop out, warm yourself on the hot granite slabs.

Getting to Horse Meadow is part of the fun. Pass McNally's Hamburger Stand near Fairview Campground on your way north of Kernville. You're into the wilderness now, so stock up while you can. Here, the canyon narrows, and you see cliffs of metamorphic rock colored by chartreuse lichen. Notice the tailings from Fairview Mine across the river. This is gold country. Pass Roads End (this was the road's end until 1939) and soon enough you turn right on Sherman Pass Road.

Sherman Pass Road heads up past buck brush, mountain mahogany, and fremontia, into chaparral with gray and pinyon pine, and finally, into Jeffrey pine, black oak, cedar, and white fir as you turn right on Cherry Hill Road. It's about 10 miles up to Horse Meadow Campground, past Alder and Brush Creeks, then Poison Meadow (note the dispersed camping sites, which require a fire permit). At the junction with Horse Meadow Road, go right 1.3 miles and you're in a tent-camping paradise.

The campground has two loops. The right loop is for tent camping only and runs along a hill above

> *This is my favorite tent campground. It's difficult to get up here, but it's worth it for the beauty and solitude.*

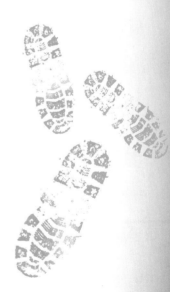

RATINGS

Beauty: ☆ ☆ ☆ ☆ ☆
Privacy: ☆ ☆
Spaciousness: ☆ ☆ ☆
Quiet: ☆ ☆ ☆ ☆
Security: ☆ ☆ ☆
Cleanliness: ☆ ☆ ☆ ☆

ADDRESS:	Horse Meadow Campground Sequoia National Forest Cannell Meadow Ranger District 105 Whitney Road, P.O. Box 9 Kernville, CA 93238
OPERATED BY:	U.S. Forest Service
INFORMATION:	(559) 784-1500; www .fs.fed.us/r5/sequoia
OPEN:	Memorial Day– mid October
SITES:	41 total; 26 for tents; 15 for RVs up to 22 feet long
EACH SITE HAS:	Picnic table, fireplace, water (phone ahead to make sure)
ASSIGNMENT:	First come, first served; no reservations
REGISTRATION:	At entrance
FACILITIES:	Vault toilets
PARKING:	At site
FEE:	$5
ELEVATION:	7,600 feet
RESTRICTIONS:	*Pets:* On leash only *Fires:* In fireplaces *Alcohol:* No restrictions *Vehicles:* Trailers not recommended

Salmon Creek and the meadow. The left loop is for tenters and small RVs. The last time I was there in July, most of the folks were tent campers. The narrow ascents up Sherman Pass and Cherry Hill Roads deter RVs and trailers. And, once you're up here, it's a long, long way down for supplies. There is good water (phone the Ranger Station before coming to make sure), but no trash bins. Haul out your garbage.

Horse Meadow is a good place to bring children. The campground loops are fine for biking, and Salmon Creek offers good trout fishing, but it's not wild and dangerous like the Kern. There are many easy hikes around the meadow, including several along Salmon Creek to some good dipping pools.

To find the upper bathing pools, go to the south side of the Horse Meadow Campground's main loop and find the trail that parallels the creek. Walk east along the left bank of the creek. Cross a spur road over Salmon Creek and keep climbing, follow the creek, and you'll come to the pools.

To visit the downstream pools, walk back past the camp entrance and go left down Salmon Falls Trail. Follow the signed trail from the parking lot and skirt the meadow. When the trail crosses Salmon Creek on a big log and goes left around a rocky butte, don't follow it. Instead, head west down the right side of the creek. The trail meanders along over rocky areas, bypassing clumps of willows, and leads you past some prime pools for dipping. The water is frigid, but the sun is blazing hot. This is heaven!

For a major hike, go back to the big log crossing Salmon Creek. With a backpack filled with soda and sandwiches, head around the rocky butte toward the Salmon Creek Falls. The trail skirts the meadow and then heads into the woods. It crosses canyons while following the south side of Salmon Creek through purple lupine country with monks hood, larkspur, and red bugler. Down by the creek, you'll see willows and dogwood.

The trail continues down to the north side of Salmon Creek and ends with a view of the Greenhorn Mountains. Those more agile than me can rock-hop down to the creek where there are more wonderful

MAP

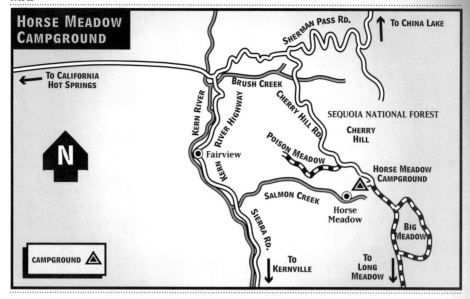

HORSE MEADOW CAMPGROUND

← TO CALIFORNIA HOT SPRINGS

SHERMAN PASS RD.

↑ TO CHINA LAKE

BRUSH CREEK

KERN RIVER

KERN RIVER HIGHWAY

CHERRY HILL RD.

SEQUOIA NATIONAL FOREST

CHERRY HILL

POISON MEADOW

Fairview

HORSE MEADOW CAMPGROUND

SALMON CREEK

SIERRA RD.

Horse Meadow

BIG MEADOW

CAMPGROUND ⛺

TO KERNVILLE

TO LONG MEADOW

pools for bathing. Just beyond them, you'll find the top of Salmon Creek Falls.

GETTING THERE

From L.A., take I-5 north to CA 99. Pass Bakersfield and take CA 178 east to Lake Isabella. Take CA 155 to Wofford Heights. Bear right to Kernville. Drive north on Sierra Way 19.4 miles and turn right on Sherman Pass Road, signed "Highway 395-Black Rock Ranger Station." Drive 6 miles, turn right on Cherry Hill Road, signed "Horse Meadow–Big Meadow." Drive 9.1 miles on the (sometimes dirt) road to the signed campground-entrance road on the right.

GPS COORDINATES

UTM Zone (WGS84) 11S

Easting [tk]

Northing [tk]

Latitude N[tk]

Longtitude W[tk]

30
LOWER
PEPPERMINT
CAMPGROUND

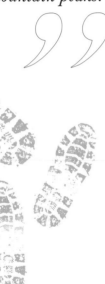

> *The Lower Peppermint area is astonishingly beautiful, with waterslides, waterfalls, and mountain peaks.*

LOWER **PEPPERMINT SITS SMACK** dab in the middle of great Northern Sierra camping near the spectacular scenery of Dome Rock and The Needles. On your way, obtain a fire permit because it increases your camping possibilities a hundredfold. You can get one from Greenhorn Ranger Station on CA 155, at Lake Isabella, a few miles east of Bakersfield, or at Cannell Meadow Ranger Station in Kernville. The free permit allows you to camp almost anywhere in Sequoia National Forest.

Sequoia National Forest calls this dispersed camping, meaning you can camp anywhere not posted off-limits. For example, around Lloyd Meadow Road dozens of old logging roads or turnoffs allow you to drive a few hundred yards and camp in a private area. Of course, you'll be expected to follow the forest's regulations—cart out your garbage, dig cat holes for bodily waste, and burn your toilet paper. Try not to leave any traces of your visit.

Buy groceries in Lake Isabella or Kernville. Once you get on Lloyd Meadows Road, there are no supplies available except beer, soda, and small bags of ice at the Johnsondale R-Ranch (turn off Parker Pass Drive 0.6 miles east of the Lloyd Meadows Road). You'll pass a cowboy guard at the gate; tell him you want to shop at the store, and he'll wave you on. The R-Ranch is a private campground. The lifetime membership fee gives access to cabins, horses, RVs, trails, etc.

Winding Lloyd Meadows Road passes through pine, white fir, cedar, and oak where there is water, and manzanita, fremontia, and digger pine where it's dry. Note turnoffs to the numbered Fire Safe Area Camps, which offer good camping (a fire permit is required to camp in Fire Safe Areas, as in all dispersed areas). During dry spells dispersed camping is confined to these areas only.

RATINGS

Beauty: ✿ ✿ ✿ ✿
Privacy: ✿ ✿ ✿ ✿
Spaciousness: ✿ ✿ ✿ ✿
Quiet: ✿ ✿ ✿ ✿ ✿
Security: ✿ ✿ ✿ ✿
Cleanliness: ✿ ✿ ✿ ✿ ✿

Lower Peppermint Campground is a small, pretty campground mostly frequented by tent campers. Boy Scouts from nearby Camp Whitsett maintain Lower Peppermint in return for the user fees on their own camp. The sites that back up to the creek are lovely.

For a great hike and swim, scramble down the bluff to the foot of the falls. Stop and swim there, or bear left along the creek until you strike a trail that takes you east. It forks south to another area of rocky pools and cascades perfect for picnicking, swimming, and sunbathing.

However, the water runs stronger than it seems, and the wet rocks by the stream are slick. The dry granite slabs above are just as bad. The granite decomposes, and the little dry bits are like ball bearings.

Another good water hike leads to the Alder Slabs. Wear clothes you don't care about, because this trip involves sliding down water chutes into cold pools on your behind. It's fun! Backtrack south on Lloyd Meadows Road and park by gated Sequoia National Forest Road 22S83. Walk north on the dirt road and then turn right down a path to Alder Creek.

Alternately, drive north from Lower Peppermint Campground to see The Needles. These amazing rock formations are crystals formed under pressure from molten rock. Pushed up, The Needles cooled along vertical master joints. Ice and erosion have done the rest. Farther north, see the Freeman Creek Grove of sequoias. En route, investigate the little intersecting roads for good future camping sites. In the dead of summer, you might want to be near water, but in the late spring, this area is so beautiful it doesn't matter where you camp—you'll be blown away by the sight of all the flowers.

Bring a saw for wood gathering, and don't forget a trowel for cat holes. I often bring a leaf rake with a sawed-off handle for clearing debris around the picnic tables and fire rings, and a shovel for fire control and digging out if the car gets stuck.

KEY INFORMATION

ADDRESS:	Lower Peppermint Campground Sequoia National Forest Tule River Ranger District 32588 CA 190 Springville, CA 93265
OPERATED BY:	U.S. Forest Service
INFORMATION:	(559) 539-2607 or (559) 784-1500; www.fs.fed.us/r5/sequoia
OPEN:	May 15– November15 (weather permitting)
SITES:	19
EACH SITE HAS:	Picnic table, fireplace
ASSIGNMENT:	First come, first served; no reservations
REGISTRATION:	At entrance
FACILITIES:	Vault toilets, water
PARKING:	At site
FEE:	$14
ELEVATION:	5,300 feet
RESTRICTIONS:	*Pets:* Allowed *Fires:* In fireplaces *Alcohol:* No restrictions *Vehicles:* Trailers not recommended

MAP

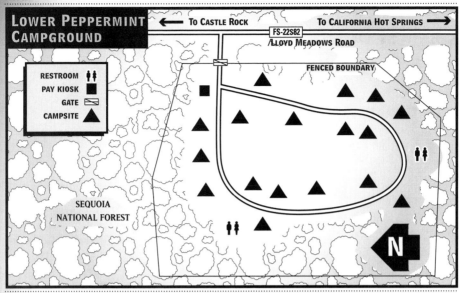

GETTING THERE

From L.A., take I-5 north
over the Tejon Pass to CA 99.
Drive north on CA 99 past
Bakersfield. Take CA 178 east
to Lake Isabella. Take CA
155 to Wofford Heights. Bear
right to Kernville. From
Kernville, drive north on
Sierra Way 19.4 miles and
turn left on Parker Pass
Drive. It is 4.9 miles to the
right-hand turn onto Lloyd
Meadows Road (Forest Ser-
vice Road 22S82). Drive
north 13.4 miles to Lower
Peppermint Campground.
Camp 6 is a few hundred
yards north on the right.

GPS COORDINATES

UTM Zone (WGS84) 11S

Easting 365741

Northing 3992329

Latitude N 36° 03' 59"

Longtitude W 118° 29' 27"

31
MINARET FALLS CAMPGROUND

MINARET FALLS CAMPGROUND is the prettiest in a string of beautiful, popular campgrounds on the Upper San Joaquin River west of Mammoth Mountain. When you drive down the dirt road into the campground, silvery Minaret Falls leaps out at you. Even in late September, on my last visit, the water cascaded down the mountainside like streams of crystal.

Right away, my wife and I drove into a campsite with a clean and soft tent pitch shrouded by trees. Through the willows we could see the riverbank and the falls.

We drove a few miles up the road to Red's Meadow store and café to buy worms and salmon eggs for trout fishing. A little bear was raiding the back room of the store, but the clerk and a tourist scared him away. A dog lunged at the end of his leash, barking at the curious animal as he scurried off. We learned that the original Red was a gold miner who turned to tourism when the Depression and falling gold prices drove him out of business. His pack station at Red's Meadow was one of the first tourist draws in the Mammoth area.

We hiked the 1.25 miles down to Rainbow Falls along with a passel of other folks. We took the rough stairs down to the exquisite falls and stood in the spray. A rainbow arced through the mist.

We hiked back through an area of firs, lodgepoles, and Jeffrey pines, scarred like most of Devil's Postpile National Monument by a 1992 wildfire. Following the fire, rangers walked through the burn to assess the damage, and charred trees crashed down around them. It wasn't safe to walk there for months.

Back at the Minaret Campground we floated salmon eggs and earthworms down the river and caught six trout. My wife wrapped them in aluminum

> *The prettiest in a string of beautiful, popular campgrounds on the Upper San Joaquin River.*

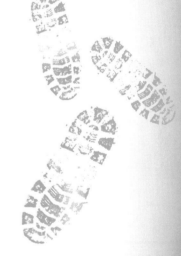

RATINGS

Beauty: ✩ ✩ ✩ ✩ ✩
Privacy: ✩ ✩ ✩
Spaciousness: ✩ ✩ ✩ ✩ ✩
Quiet: ✩ ✩ ✩ ✩ ✩
Security: ✩ ✩ ✩ ✩ ✩
Cleanliness: ✩ ✩ ✩ ✩

KEY INFORMATION

ADDRESS:	Minaret Falls Campground Inyo National Forest 351 Pacu Lane Suite 200 Bishop, CA 93514
OPERATED BY:	U.S. Forest Service
INFORMATION:	(760) 873-2400; www .fs.fed.us/r5/inyo
OPEN:	June 15– September 19
SITES:	28
EACH SITE HAS:	Picnic table, fireplace
ASSIGNMENT:	First come, first served; no reservations
REGISTRATION:	At entrance
FACILITIES:	Water, chemical toilets
PARKING:	At site
FEE:	$16
ELEVATION:	7,600 feet
RESTRICTIONS:	*Pets:* On leash only *Fires:* In fireplace *Alcohol:* No restrictions *Vehicles:* RVs up to 22 feet *Other:* No dispersed camping in this area; 14-day stay limit. *Note:* To reduce vehicle traffic into the Devil's Postpile area, a shuttle bus system has been implemented. Campers pay a one-time fee exemption. Stop at the Mammoth Lakes visitor center (on the right side of CA 203 on the way into Mammoth Lakes) or the Adventure Center (at the ski area) for more information.

foil with herbs and cooked them over the campfire. It was a gorgeous night. The Southern Sierras have hundreds of shooting stars.

Sleeping that night in our tent, I heard the rustle of a visitor—a bear. He ran away when I got up. I inspected the damage. My two treasured inflatable Basic Designs sinks, which my wife and I use to wash the dishes, were ruined. The bear had bitten a big hole in each of them. To add insult to injury, he also bit into my plastic collapsible water jug. Were these acts of rancor, or did he think they were full of food?

A neighbor came over. The bear had tried to open the hatch of his Nissan Z; the telltale paw marks gave the intruder away. I told him about my sinks. He recommended wiping sinks, picnic tables, and cooler tops each night with bleach. Bears like soap; bears like everything except bleach. I went back to my sleeping bag and heard the bear slouch through the camp again.

The next morning we walked north along the river and crossed on a log at the end of the campground. There's a short trail to the foot of Minaret Falls. We bushwhacked up to the top of the falls and dipped in some nice pools.

Later, we hiked up to Shadow Lake. It's no easy climb (round-trip is about 7 miles), but you'll agree it's worth it when you see beautiful blue Shadow Lake against huge, craggy Mount Ritter. To find the trailhead, drive back toward Mammoth from the Minaret Falls Campground. Take the road to Agnew Meadows Campground. About 0.3 miles in, you'll find trailhead parking with toilets and drinking water. Follow the signs to Shadow Lake, through another parking lot and across a creek to another trail junction at about 1 mile. To the left is Red's Meadow. To the right is Shadow Lake. With Mammoth Mountain at your back, climb up past Olaine Lake, cross the San Joaquin River on a wooden bridge, and hoof it up the canyon wall to Shadow Lake. You'll find good fishing, so bring your fishing gear and bait.

Minaret Falls Campground is popular. Be sure to phone rangers ahead of time to make sure it's open and to see how crowded it will be. Try to plan a trip before or after the prime summertime season and arrive on

MAP

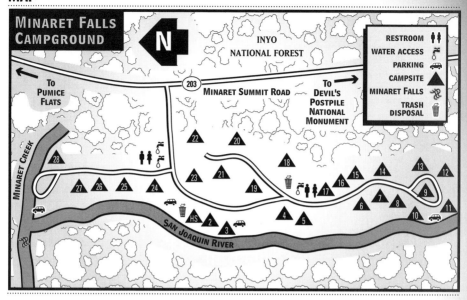

MINARET FALLS CAMPGROUND

N

INYO NATIONAL FOREST

To PUMICE FLATS

203 MINARET SUMMIT ROAD

To DEVIL'S POSTPILE NATIONAL MONUMENT

RESTROOM
WATER ACCESS
PARKING
CAMPSITE
MINARET FALLS
TRASH DISPOSAL

MINARET CREEK

SAN JOAQUIN RIVER

Thursday if you want to spend the weekend. The area is so popular that during the summer, hikers (not campers) are required to park their cars at the Mammoth Ski Resort and take an intravalley shuttle down.

You have 30 minutes from the time you occupy a campsite to pay. Park your car at the first empty campsite you find and use that 30 minutes to walk around and see if you like another site better. If you find one, leave something on the picnic table and go move your car.

GETTING THERE

From L.A., take I-5 north to CA 14. Take CA 14 north to US 395 near Inyokern. Continue north on US 395 for 123 miles to Bishop. Continue another 37 miles on US 395 to Mammoth Lakes. From Mammoth Lakes, drive 16 miles west on CA 203 (Minaret Summit Road) to the campground.

GPS COORDINATES

UTM Zone (WGS84) 11S
Easting 316137
Northing 4167850
Latitude N 37° 38' 22"
Longtitude W 119° 05' 02"

32
MORAINE
CAMPGROUND

A grand canyon and a pretty valley combine for sublime scenery.

EVERYBODY BUT **ANDREW MARVELL,** the 17th-century English poet, loves mountains. He called them "ill-designed excrescences" (abnormal growths). Of course, Marvell was a flatlander who never visited Kings Canyon National Park.

William Brewer did, however, and waxed eloquently about the Moraine Campground area in 1864:

> *This is the grandest canyon I have ever seen. A pretty valley or flat half-a-mile wide lies along the river covered with trees. On both sides rise tremendous granite precipices, of every shape, often nearly perpendicular, rising from 2,500 feet to above 4,000 feet. They did not form a continuous wall, but rose in high points, with canyons coming down here and there, and with fissures, gashes, and gorges. The whole scene was sublime.*

It is sublime. And it's the mountains—not the standard national-park-issue campground—that elicit this feeling. You would not come to Moraine Campground if it were not below Sentinel Ridge and Monarch Divide. However, just the spectacular drive justifies a visit. Take the wide and well-banked, convict-built CA 180 all the way in from Fresno. Coming over the rise to see the gorge and the mountains behind it takes your breath away. Then, circle down and follow the river to Cedar Grove and Moraine Campground.

There is a store at Cedar Grove that sells ice, beverages, and some food, and there is a cafeteria for folks tired of camp cooking. There are hot showers and a Laundromat. For an ice cream or a sandwich, stop at Kings Canyon Lodge on the way in or out, approximately halfway between Grants Grove and Cedar Grove. The charming lodge is rustic but beautiful, with flower beds mixed in with old, rusted mining equipment. The little cabins were authentic dwellings of early-20th-century miners.

RATINGS

Beauty: ☆ ☆ ☆ ☆ ☆
Privacy: ☆ ☆ ☆
Spaciousness: ☆ ☆ ☆ ☆
Quiet: ☆ ☆ ☆ ☆ ☆
Security: ☆ ☆ ☆ ☆
Cleanliness: ☆ ☆ ☆ ☆ ☆

A little farther on is Boyden Cavern. I plunked down my $10 for the guided tour. Native Americans avoided the place, feeling that bad spirits lived there. I can see why. I swallowed hard when the guide turned off the lights and described the mile or so of solid granite over our heads. The children on the tour were thrilled.

Another fun activity for children at Cedar Grove is a horse ride at Cedar Grove Pack Station. Here, you can arrange anything from a one-hour ride to a week-long trip into the backcountry. They offer kiddy rides as well. If you come to camp and want to arrange a more elaborate ride, it's best to phone ahead and make reservations. Call (559) 565-3464.

The river was running too fast for much fishing the last time I was at Cedar Grove in August. However, the cowboys at the stables told me you could do all right if you knew where to fish. "Where's that?" I asked, but they laughed and wouldn't disclose any information.

Upriver from Moraine, there are several parking areas where you can pull over and walk down to the river. The second or third areas access a part of the river where the current runs languidly even at flood tide. I wonder if this is the cowboy fishing hole? I got my lure wet, but there were no trout takers.

Farther on, past the bridge on the left, you'll find the beginning of the Cedar Grove Motor Nature Trail, a dirt road that heads back to Cedar Grove Village across the North Fork Kings River. It passes several great places to park and hang out down by the water.

You can't leave Cedar Grove without hiking up to Mist Falls. The trailhead is at Roads End, about 6 miles from the Ranger Station in Cedar Grove. Right away, you'll cross Copper Creek, near the site of a former Native American village. Look carefully and you'll find flakes of obsidian, which Native Americans used to make weapons and tools. There was a store here once, and John Muir swore by the pies the owner's wife, Viola, made. About 2 miles in, head uphill following the river. On your left is Buck Peak (8,776 feet), and The Sphinx (9,146 feet) is behind you. See if you can sort out the ponderosa, Jeffrey, and sugar pines. To the

KEY INFORMATION

ADDRESS:	Moraine Campground Kings Canyon National Park 47050 Generals Highway Three Rivers, CA 93271-9700
OPERATED BY:	National Park Service
INFORMATION:	(559) 565-3341; www.nps.gov/seki
OPEN:	Late May–mid November (weather permitting)
SITES:	120
EACH SITE HAS:	Picnic table, fire pit, bear box
ASSIGNMENT:	First come, first served; no reservations
REGISTRATION:	At entrance
FACILITIES:	Water, flush toilets, coin-operated showers, wheelchair-accessible sites
PARKING:	At site
FEE:	$18
ELEVATION:	4,600 feet
RESTRICTIONS:	*Pets:* On leash only *Fires:* In fire pits only, may be restricted during high fire danger *Alcohol:* No restrictions *Vehicles:* 1 per site maximum *Other:* 6 campers per site maximum; 14-day stay limit

MAP

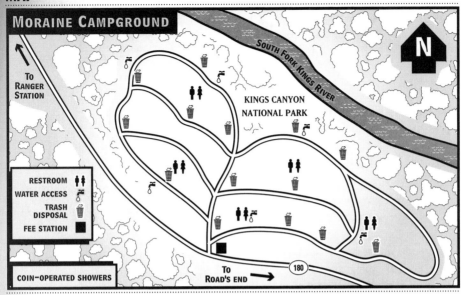

MORAINE CAMPGROUND

To RANGER STATION

SOUTH FORK KINGS RIVER

N

KINGS CANYON NATIONAL PARK

RESTROOM
WATER ACCESS
TRASH DISPOSAL
FEE STATION

COIN-OPERATED SHOWERS

To ROAD'S END →

180

GETTING THERE

From L.A., take I-5 north over the Tejon Pass to CA 99. Drive north past Bakersfield 104 miles to Fresno. Go east on CA 180 to Kings Canyon National Park. Follow CA 180 for 29 miles to Cedar Grove Village. From Cedar Grove Village drive east on CA 180 for 1 mile to the campground.

GPS COORDINATES

UTM Zone (WGS84) 11S
Easting 351872
Northing 4072406
Latitude N 36° 47' 09"
Longtitude W 118° 39' 36"

east, don't miss the waterfall on Gardiner Creek. Soon enough, you'll reach Mist Falls, and the sight is worth the climb.

The best time to visit Moraine Campground at Cedar Grove is in the spring. It's cool enough then to hike comfortably all day long, and the crowds haven't begun to arrive in droves, as in August. Still, Kings Canyon National Park is beautiful any month of the year.

33
PRINCESS
CAMPGROUND

YOU'LL LOVE **PRINCESS CAMPGROUND** just like you love a golden retriever for being a basic, good dog. Princess is a campground's campground. Set under the shade of second-growth sequoias and pines, Princess is covered on one flank by a shimmering alpine meadow. The campsites are private and level, and everything is well maintained and clean.

Hume Lake, 3 miles down the road, is a big draw for anybody with a vinyl water toy or a fishing rod. A huge Christian campground occupies one end of the lake's shoreline. Dammed up by lumber folks, Hume Lake supplied the water for the flume that scooted timber down to Sanger in the San Joaquin Valley 54 miles away. Flumes work on the same principle as water slides: water reduces friction.

Unlike the water in the mountain streams, Hume Lake warms up enough that you can actually swim without turning gelid. A path encircles the lake, and you can find your own grassy beach spot. Air mattresses or inexpensive blow-up boats are big hits. I saw people catching edible-sized fish as well.

A choice spot is Sandy Cove Beach. Coming down from CA 180, pass Hume Lake Campground and follow the road around past the Powder Canyon Picnic Area, through the Hume Lake Christian Camp, and along Lakeshore Drive to Sandy Cove Beach. This is a fun and safe place to swim, where the trill of youthful swimmers' voices resounds. Adults with more secluded sunbathing in mind can follow Landslide Creek up to find a private spot. The road that heads south to Generals Highway follows the creek most of the way.

Princess is regarded as an overflow campground for Hume Lake, but I find it offers much better camping. It's quieter and cleaner, and because you have to walk downhill to the lake from Hume Lake

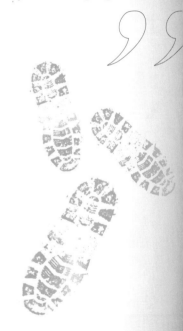

> *This campground has everything—big trees, warm lakes, and fantastic gorge views.*

RATINGS

Beauty: ✪ ✪ ✪ ✪
Privacy: ✪ ✪ ✪ ✪
Spaciousness: ✪ ✪ ✪ ✪
Quiet: ✪ ✪ ✪
Security: ✪ ✪ ✪
Cleanliness: ✪ ✪ ✪ ✪

KEY INFORMATION

ADDRESS:	Princess Campground Sequoia National Forest Hume Lake Ranger District 35860 East Kings Canyon Road Dunlap, CA 93621
OPERATED BY:	California Land Management
INFORMATION:	(559) 784-1500; www .fs.fed.us/r5/sequoia
OPEN:	May–October
SITES:	20 tent; 70 sites for RVs up to 32 feet
EACH SITE HAS:	Picnic table, fireplace
ASSIGNMENT:	Some sites require reservations; others are first come, first served.
REGISTRATION:	At entrance; reserve by phone, (877) 444-6777, or online, www.reserveusa .com, 3 days in advance.
FACILITIES:	Water, vault toilets
PARKING:	At site
FEE:	$17–$19, plus $1.50 reservation fee; must pay national-park entrance fee
ELEVATION:	5,900 feet
RESTRICTIONS:	*Pets:* On leash only *Fires:* In fireplace *Alcohol:* No restrictions *Vehicles:* RVs up to 32 feet

Campground, you might as well drive down from Princess. At least up there you won't suffer the incessant camp counselors' whistles in the morning. And the added 700 feet of elevation at Princess cuts down on the bugs and the dust.

The Indian Basin Grove Trail is an easy one-hour hike, starting about half a mile west of the Princess Campground entrance. You can walk there from Princess or take a car and park in a turnout just west of the road. The trail follows Forest Service Road 13S50 north through ponderosas and cedars. Look for the sequoia stumps, then for the second-generation sequoias growing back. After a mile or so, pass Forest Service Road 13S07, which could take you back to Princess Campground, but persevere and follow the road north to a ridge. When the road turns east, find the trail in a patch of manzanita. The trail continues north to a point overlooking Kings Canyon.

Another good hike is to the Boole Tree. Drive west on CA 180 to Forest Service Road 13S55, then drive 2.7 miles to the trailhead parking lot. Follow the signed trail. It's an easy 2-mile trip in and out. Be sure to see the tree—it's an incredible sight. Why didn't loggers ever cut it down? Nobody knows, but some say Frank Boole, general manager of the Sanger Lumber Company, spared the tree as a tribute to himself.

Just up the road is Grant Grove, with more incredible sequoias. One tree actually antedates Christ by 1,500 years. Sequoias do not die of old age; they are the closest we'll get to eternity until we go to our own rewards. The short walk out to Panoramic Point is fun, especially at sunset.

At Grant Grove Village you can buy ice, soda, and beer. Many families stay at Princess Campground. The last time I was there, I camped next to a schoolteacher and his herd of children. He was an erudite chap and taught his wee ones some games originating with the Monachi and Yokut Native Americans. Their favorite involved guessing who on the opposing team held a rock beneath an all-concealing blanket.

There are no bear boxes at Princess Campground, but there are black bears. You must be careful

MAP

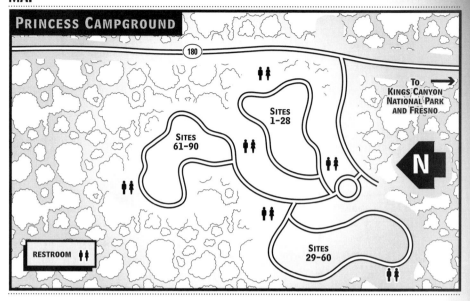

PRINCESS CAMPGROUND

180

TO
KINGS CANYON
NATIONAL PARK
AND FRESNO

SITES
1-28

SITES
61-90

N

SITES
29-60

RESTROOM

with your food. As soon as you eat, take the trash to the bins. Conceal your cooler in your car. The bears recognize coolers and know their purpose. Don't leave anything in your tent that has a strong odor, such as sunscreen, lipstick, skin cream, etc. Rangers shoot bears when they become repeat food raiders, so be cool and save a bear.

GETTING THERE

From L.A., take I-5 north over the Tejon Pass to CA 99. Drive north past Bakersfield 104 miles to Fresno. Go east on CA 180 to Kings Canyon National Park. Follow CA 180 to Grant Grove. From Grant Grove in Kings Canyon National Park, drive 6 miles north to Princess Campground on the right.

GPS COORDINATES

UTM Zone (WGS84) 11S
Easting 326820
Northing 4074841
Latitude N 36° 18' 13"
Longtitude W 118° 56' 29"

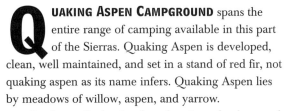

> *Come in the fall for autumn leaves and in the summer for hiking and mountain biking.*

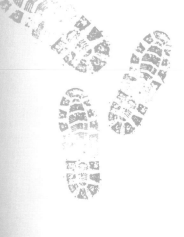

QUAKING **A**SPEN **C**AMPGROUND spans the entire range of camping available in this part of the Sierras. Quaking Aspen is developed, clean, well maintained, and set in a stand of red fir, not quaking aspen as its name infers. Quaking Aspen lies by meadows of willow, aspen, and yarrow.

Ponderosa Lodge is a fun place to grab a beer and chili or to pick up ice, but don't plan on shopping there. Springville is the last port of call for supplies. This pretty little town in Tule River country has just about everything you'll need. Before Jedediah Smith trapped beaver here in 1827, the Yaudanchis (a sub-tribe of the Yokut) lived in the foothills during the winter and trekked to the mountains to gather food in the summer. By 1857, the Yaudanchis were history.

Settlers poured into the area. John Nelson forged his way up the canyon of the Middle Fork of the Tule River (CA 190 east of Springville today) and filed a claim on property that is now Camp Nelson. Springville (named for the soda springs in the area) was the site of a mill that processed the raw timber that was hauled down by horse- and mule-team wagons from the higher reaches of what is today Sequoia National Forest. Logging continued into the early 1900s, when the Porterville Northeastern Railroad built a spur into Springville. Then, finished lumber, citrus fruits, and apples could be shipped to the valley below.

Now, citrus orchards dot the lower foothills leading into town along CA 190. Ranching operations spread across wide-open parcels of oak- and buckeye-studded hills. Apples are grown farther up on the cooler, protected slopes, merging into the manzanita, black oak, cedar, and pine. Logging continues under the supervision of the Sequoia National Forest.

RATINGS

Beauty: ✪ ✪ ✪ ✪ ✪
Privacy: ✪ ✪ ✪ ✪
Spaciousness: ✪ ✪ ✪ ✪
Quiet: ✪ ✪ ✪ ✪
Security: ✪ ✪ ✪ ✪ ✪
Cleanliness: ✪ ✪ ✪ ✪ ✪

Between Quaking Aspen Campground and Ponderosa Lodge, note the actual quaking aspens that give the campground its name. These slender trees have light bark and roundish leaves. Vivid green in spring and bright gold in fall, the leaves quiver at the least breath of breeze.

The good bathing holes on Peppermint Creek are downstream from the campground about a quarter of a mile. Stick to the south side of the creek, because it's hard to cross over from the other side. The wet rocks are extremely slippery. Don't even think of crossing on them. Find a place with a sandy bottom before you try getting in the water. Also, watch out for the granite slabs on the banks. Their surface decomposes, leaving slippery bits of rock.

A great hike is out to the Needles Lookout. It's only a 4-mile round-trip of pretty easy walking, but plan on making a day of it. Take lunch. The dirt road to the trailhead takes off to the east about 0.5 miles south of Ponderosa Lodge. Drive 2.8 miles in and park. The trail begins at the east end of the parking lot. Note the small purple flowers along the trail. They are called pennyroyals (*Mentha pulegium*) and are used to make mint tea. Pennyroyals are not local, however; they are natives of Europe brought in by the forty-niners.

Along the trail, look north to Kaweah peaks and Mount Whitney and northeast to the Kern Plateau peaks of Kern and Olancha. Then, keep an eye out for the lookout on top of the westernmost Needle—it's a fire tower manned in fire season.

Believe me, the view is worth the slog up the switchback ladders to the catwalk. Talk to the fire watcher if he is on duty. This place can get hairy. In storms, the lookout is frequently struck by lightning. In fact, the fire watcher has a special stool fitted with glass insulators that he sits on when there is lightning striking nearby!

The camping at Quaking Aspen Campground is especially beautiful in the fall with the turning of the leaves. I enjoyed Quaking Aspen in the summer as well. It's a very gracious place and is the birthplace of my famous one-pot Hungarian potato–hot dog stew.

KEY INFORMATION

ADDRESS: Quaking Aspen Campground Sequoia National Forest Tule River Ranger District 32588 CA 190 Springville, CA 93265

OPERATED BY: U.S. Forest Service

INFORMATION: (559) 784-1500 or (559) 539-2607; www.recreation.gov

OPEN: April–November

SITES: 32

EACH SITE HAS: Picnic table, fireplace

ASSIGNMENT: Some sites require reservations; others are first come, first served.

REGISTRATION: At entrance; reserve by phone, (877) 444-6777, or online, www.reserveusa .com.

FACILITIES: Water, vault toilets

PARKING: At site

FEE: $17, plus $1.50 reservation fee

ELEVATION: 7,000 feet

RESTRICTIONS: *Pets:* On leash only *Fires:* In fireplaces *Alcohol:* No restrictions *Vehicles:* RVs up to 27 feet *Other:* 2 wheelchair-accessible sites; 14-day stay limit

MAP

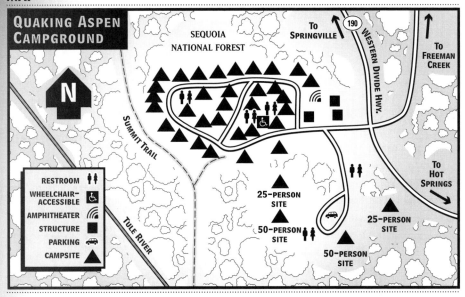

GETTING THERE

From L.A., take I-5 north over the Tejon Pass to CA 99. Drive north on CA 99 past Bakersfield. Take CA 65 north to Porterville. Go east 17 miles on CA 190 to Springville. From Springville, drive 23.3 miles east on CA 190 to Quaking Aspen Campground on the right.

GPS COORDINATES

UTM Zone (WGS84) 11S
Easting 360852
Northing 3995818
Latitude N 36° 07' 17"
Longtitude W 118° 32' 46"

Sauté diced onions in a little oil in a pot. Add quartered potatoes and hot paprika. Stir and cover. Simmer until potatoes are almost done, then add hot dogs and simmer. Eat. Food good.

35 RANCHERIA CAMPGROUND

RANCHERIA **C**AMPGROUND **ON** Huntington Lake is big, handsome, and noisy. The acoustics around camp on the pine-shored lake are such that you can hear a mouse belch at dusk from the south shore. You'll hear folks laughing on boats at the nearby marina, outboards putting on fishing skiffs, chaps hammering siding on cottages by the town of Lake Shore, and the occasional Fire Service helicopter flyby. It feels like one big, beautiful neighborhood.

The campground has been around for a long time, and the sites are screened by pine and brush. Many are walk-ins along the lake, allowing you to pitch your tent right on the shore. Folks with boats can tie them to a root next to their campsite. The beach slopes gently into the water, which makes for good wading. There are sites back in the woods, too, for people who want to avoid all the aquatic activity.

Perched on the edge of the wilderness, Huntington Lake is a good first camp for anyone heading farther in to Thomas A. Edison Lake (aka Edison Lake) or Florence Lake. You'll find last-chance shopping at the country store in Lake Shore and information at the Ranger Station. There's a good chance that you will want to settle in at Rancheria and forget the hairy drive up over Kaiser Pass.

The lakes in this region comprise the Big Creek hydroelectric project, owned by Southern California Edison. Water runs from Edison and Florence lakes before flowing into Huntington Lake and on to Shaver Lake, turning turbines along the way.

C. B. Shaver was the first to use the power of water here when he built a millpond to saw lumber before floating it down a 40-mile flume to Clovis. When the lumber gave out, the power company moved in and built dams and reservoirs.

> *Though sometimes crowded, lakeside Rancheria Campground offers solid, safe tent camping.*

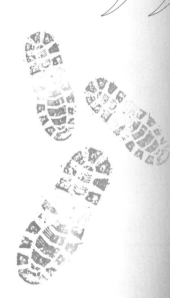

RATINGS

Beauty: ✿ ✿ ✿ ✿
Privacy: ✿ ✿ ✿ ✿
Spaciousness: ✿ ✿ ✿ ✿
Quiet: ✿ ✿ ✿ ✿ ✿
Security: ✿ ✿ ✿ ✿
Cleanliness: ✿ ✿ ✿ ✿ ✿

ADDRESS: Rancheria Campground Sierra National Forest Supervisor's Office P.O. Box 559 Prather, CA 93651

OPERATED BY: California Land Management

INFORMATION: (559) 297-0706 or (559) 893-2111; www.fs.fed.us/r5/sierra; California road conditions: (800) 427-ROAD (7623); outside California, (916) 445-7623; www.dot.ca.gov/hq/roadinfo

OPEN: June–October

SITES: 149 sites (some tents only)

EACH SITE HAS: Picnic table, fire ring, parking spur

ASSIGNMENT: Reservations highly recommended

REGISTRATION: At entrance; reserve by phone, (877) 444-6777, or online, www.recreation.gov.

FACILITIES: Water, flush and vault toilets

PARKING: At or near site

FEE: $19, single site; $21, premium site, plus $1.50 reservation fee

ELEVATION: 7,000 feet

RESTRICTIONS: *Pets:* On leash only
Fires: In fireplace
Alcohol: No restrictions
Vehicles: RVs up to 40 feet
Other: Camp in color-coded sites—yellow for tents, blue for RVs up to 20 feet, white for RVs up to 30 feet, red for RVs up to 40 feet; 14-day stay limit

For a power company, water in a reservoir is like money in the bank. It provides cheap, clean, reliable power that can be used almost immediately. As long as the lakes are full, the vacationing public is happy. But, nothing is uglier than an empty lake.

You can rent boats at the marina across from Rancheria Campground. Or, visit in the winter and ski at nearby Sierra Summit Ski Resort on Chinese Peak. I found the skiing spectacular, but heard some experts complaining that the best runs were too short. Hike up to Rancheria Falls from the trailhead across the road from Rancheria Campground. Or, hike to the river pools. The trailhead is in the second parking lot of the ski resort.

There is decent shopping at Ken's Market in Shaver Lake, and you'll find beer, ice, and sundries at the friendly country store in Lake Shore. But, if you want a sirloin steak, you better bring it with you. While you're packing, it's not a bad idea to bring a pair of shoes to wear in and around the lake.

And, don't accommodate the bears! Put all edibles in your car and out of view. Bring a small bottle of bleach and wipe down your cooking gear and picnic table before turning in. Bears don't like the smell; maybe they associate it with the toilet facilities.

When I was there in September, the bears were especially active at Lower Billy Campground on the other side of Lake Shore. I spoke to a woman at the Ranger Station, who said that a bear broke into her storage shed a few nights before and ate everything but some frozen ears of corn. That was at 3:14 a.m. The next night, the bear came back at exactly 3:14 a.m. for the frozen corn.

Be sure to read the memorial on the rock by the Ranger Station. It honors a crew of airmen who died in 1944. Apparently, a B-24 bomber ran into trouble. The pilot gave the crew two options—bail out or stay with the ship and gut it out. Two men jumped and lived. The plane disappeared into the blue and was lost for a decade. Finally, in 1955, the power company lowered the water in Huntington Lake to make some repairs on the dam. The receding water revealed the

MAP

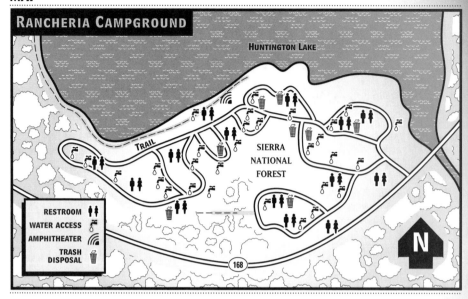

RANCHERIA CAMPGROUND

HUNTINGTON LAKE

TRAIL

SIERRA NATIONAL FOREST

RESTROOM
WATER ACCESS
AMPHITHEATER
TRASH DISPOSAL

N

168

wreckage of the missing B-24 and the bodies of the remaining crew members.

I thought of those young men as I swam in azure Huntington Lake and stood in the mist from the generator turbines by the Kaiser Pass Road. Maybe it would be better if they hadn't been found. Then, we could always think of them out there somewhere, handsome and young in sheepskin flying jackets, their faces full of promise.

GETTING THERE

From L.A., take I-5 north over the Tejon Pass to CA 99. Drive north past Bakersfield 104 miles to Fresno. Take CA 41 north to CA 168. Go northeast to Shaver Lake and head 20 miles north on CA 168. Rancheria Campground is on the left as you come to the head of Huntington Lake.

GPS COORDINATES

UTM Zone (WGS84) 11S
Easting 308244
Northing 4121519
Latitude N 37° 14' 52"
Longtitude W 119° 09' 43"

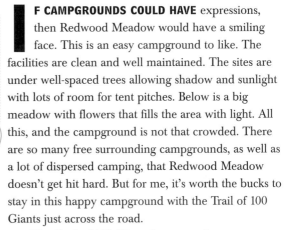

> *A happy campground with the Trail of 100 Giants and a meadow full of flowers.*

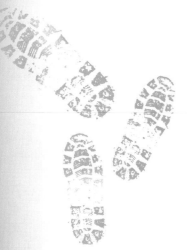

IF CAMPGROUNDS COULD HAVE expressions, then Redwood Meadow would have a smiling face. This is an easy campground to like. The facilities are clean and well maintained. The sites are under well-spaced trees allowing shadow and sunlight with lots of room for tent pitches. Below is a big meadow with flowers that fills the area with light. All this, and the campground is not that crowded. There are so many free surrounding campgrounds, as well as a lot of dispersed camping, that Redwood Meadow doesn't get hit hard. But for me, it's worth the bucks to stay in this happy campground with the Trail of 100 Giants just across the road.

The Trail of 100 Giants is a great place to get acquainted with the "Big Trees." The largest tree in the grove has a diameter of 20 feet and is 220 feet in height. The trees' ages range between 500 and 1,500 years old. These old guys were babes when the Roman Empire fell.

Back in the glacial eras, the giant sequoias (*Sequoiadendron gigantuem*) grew all over what is now the western United States. When the climate dried out, the sequoias retreated to ecological islands with abundant rainfall and runoff, where they grow mostly in granite basins or where bedrock is near the surface.

Try to burn a piece of redwood bark and you'll see how resistant it is to fire. The bark is impregnated with tannins that are resistant to both fire and insects. That allows the trees to grow very old. And, given abundant moisture, redwoods are the fastest-growing trees in the United States. Age and growth rate explain why the giant sequoias are so huge.

For years, foresters tried to protect the giant sequoia from fire. Only recently did they realize that the sequoias need fire to perpetuate. Ground fires do not burn through the bark, but the rising heat opens

RATINGS

Beauty: ✪ ✪ ✪ ✪ ✪
Privacy: ✪ ✪ ✪
Spaciousness: ✪ ✪ ✪ ✪
Quiet: ✪ ✪ ✪ ✪
Security: ✪ ✪ ✪
Cleanliness: ✪ ✪ ✪ ✪

the cones, which remain on the trees for up to 20 years. When the cones open, the seeds fall on the soft, recently burned earth. When it rains, these seeds germinate in the sunlight that shines to the ground freely through the recently burned foliage.

An interesting friend of the giant sequoia is the giant carpenter ant who makes nests in the sequoias by hollowing them out. Try not to think about the ant when you're standing under a giant sequoia, and pray for an occasional fire, since it reduces the population of the giant ants.

For bicycling, Western Divide Highway is a great option. The road is wide with no blind curves. On a weekday you'll hardly see a car. A good tour is from Redwood Meadow Campground to Ponderosa Lodge and back. The round-trip is about 24 miles. You'll bike from good clear water available at the campground to the Ponderosa Lodge's varied liquid refreshments and breakfast, lunch, and dinner choices, then back home again to the campground. On the way, a short section of dirt road takes you to Dome Rock—be sure to stop. A quick walk along an obvious path will lead you to a spectacular view. Look down and you'll see the slash of Kern Canyon. Spot The Needles, and Peppermint Creek below. What a wild, lovely vista!

Another great mountain-bike trip is down the connector road that heads left from Western Divide Highway about 3 to 4 miles from Redwood Campground. It climbs Nobe Creek basin to Windy Gap, then passes Coy Flat Campground, and ends up at Camp Nelson (about 24 miles one-way). I found the trip to be quite long, and was greatly relieved when someone in our party hitched a ride on a pickup truck back to Redwood Campground to get a relief vehicle.

Reserve a site at Redwood Meadow Campground on big weekends. I especially like sites 2 through 8, because they are off the highway and back down to the little stream. If the campground is too busy, head north a half mile on Western Divide Highway. To the right is a dirt road leading down to Long Meadow Campground, a delightful place to pitch a tent (get a fire permit from the Ranger Station—it's good for the year!).

KEY INFORMATION

ADDRESS:	Redwood Meadow Campground Sequoia National Forest Tule River Ranger District 32588 CA 190 Springville, CA 93265
OPERATED BY:	Sequoia National Forest
INFORMATION:	(559) 539-3004 or (559) 784-1500; www.fs.fed.us/r5/sequoia
OPEN:	May 15–November 15 (weather permitting)
SITES:	15
EACH SITE HAS:	Picnic table, fireplace
ASSIGNMENT:	Some sites require reservations; others are first come, first served.
REGISTRATION:	At entrance; reserve by phone, (877) 444-6777, or online, www.reserveusa.com.
FACILITIES:	Vault toilets, water (phone ahead)
PARKING:	At site
FEE:	$17, plus $1.50 reservation fee
ELEVATION:	6,500 feet
RESTRICTIONS:	*Pets:* Allowed *Fires:* In fireplaces *Alcohol:* No restrictions *Vehicles:* RVs up to 16 feet

MAP

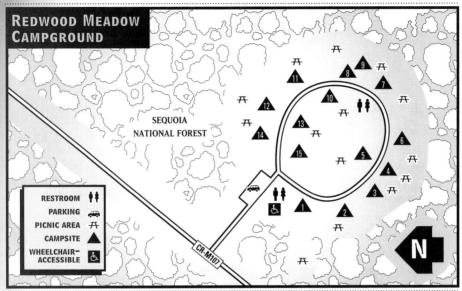

REDWOOD MEADOW CAMPGROUND

SEQUOIA NATIONAL FOREST

RESTROOM
PARKING
PICNIC AREA
CAMPSITE
WHEELCHAIR-ACCESSIBLE

CR-M107

N

GETTING THERE

From L.A., take I-5 north to CA 99. Drive north past Bakersfield. Take CA 178 east to Lake Isabella. Take CA 155 to Wofford Heights. Bear right to Kernville, and drive north on Sierra Way 19.4 miles. Turn left on Parker Pass Road. Drive 10.4 miles to Western Divide Highway. Go right, and the campground is 3 miles up on the right.

Or, try Holey Meadow Campground. Or, head back to Parker Pass Road and go east. Almost immediately, you'll find turnoffs to good dispersed camping on the right by the stream. Armed with a fire permit, you can find great camping spots anytime in this area.

GPS COORDINATES

UTM Zone (WGS84) 11S

Easting 356437

Northing 3982525

Latitude N 35° 58' 36"

Longtitude W 118° 35' 32"

37
SADDLEBAG
LAKE CAMPGROUND

*Inyo National Forest,
just east of Yosemite
National Park*

T**HE SIERRA NEVADA LANDSCAPE** is a pristine and dramatic mix of glacier-carved granite, snow-fed streams and lakes, wildflower-dotted meadows, and ancient forests; this is one of the most beautiful places in the world. At a high alpine elevation, the campground season is short, just a five-month stretch from June (sometimes later) to mid-October. Camping here is like eating the first local strawberries of spring after a winter of tasteless hothouse fruit: intense, sweet, and fleeting. It may spoil you for anyplace else.

Saddlebag Lake is one of five intimate, nonreservable Inyo National Forest campgrounds a mere 2 miles east of the Yosemite National Park entrance station at Tioga Pass. At Tioga Lake, a cluster of open sites sprawl on the lake (but also right off CA 120). Junction Campground, at the intersection of Saddlebag Lake Road and CA 120, is a short distance off both roads, but has more trees to provide privacy. Less than a mile east of Saddlebag Lake Road sits Ellery Lake, slightly downhill from CA 120. This campground has some sites well screened by shrubby willows, directly on Lee Vining Creek. Proceeding 1.6 miles up Saddlebag Lake Road, you'll find the easy-to-miss Sawmill Walk-in Campground, on the left. It's a short, level walk to a gorgeous 12-spot campground with well-spaced sites sprinkled across a rocky alpine meadow dotted with pine. At the end of Saddlebag Lake Road sits the crown jewel of the area, Saddlebag Lake, its namesake campground, and trailheads for the 20-lakes basin.

Saddlebag Lake Campground, on a hill above the lake, is reached via a steep gravel road. Although there is plenty of daytime activity down by the lake, the campground is exceptionally quiet. Sites radiate off a single loop, and the ground is somewhat sloped, but gravel tent pads provide level pitches. The premier

Perched on a knoll overlooking one of a series of jewel-like alpine lakes.

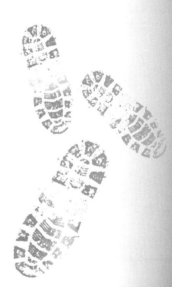

RATINGS

Beauty: ✰ ✰ ✰ ✰
Privacy: ✰ ✰ ✰
Spaciousness: ✰ ✰ ✰ ✰
Quiet: ✰ ✰ ✰ ✰ ✰
Security: ✰ ✰ ✰ ✰ ✰
Cleanliness: ✰ ✰ ✰ ✰ ✰

ADDRESS: Lee Vining Ranger Station
Inyo National Forest
P.O. Box 429
Lee Vining,
CA 93541

OPERATED BY: National Forest Service

INFORMATION: Mono Basin Scenic Area visitor center, (760) 873-2538; www.fs.fed.us/r5/inyo

OPEN: June 1–October 15 (weather permitting); if planning early- or late-season camping, call to be sure the campground is open

SITES: 20 sites for tents or RVs (no designated RV spots, hookups, or dump station)

EACH SITE HAS: Picnic table, fire ring, food storage locker

ASSIGNMENT: First come, first served; no reservations

REGISTRATION: Self-register at information station

FACILITIES: Drinking water, vault toilets

PARKING: At individual sites

FEE: $17; if arriving from the west, $20 entrance fee for Yosemite

ELEVATION: 10,087 feet

RESTRICTIONS: *Pets:* Dogs are permitted, on leash during the day and in your tent at night. *Fires:* In designated fire rings only *Alcohol:* No restrictions *Other:* 14-day stay limit

sites are 16, 18, and 19, which overlook the lake, but most of the other sites offer at least partial views to the water as well as the rugged peaks to the north. Spindly lodgepole pines offer only moderate screening between sites, but heck, everyone's looking at the lake anyway.

The lake is actually a dammed reservoir, the water from which flows into Lee Vining Creek and then down to Lee Vining, where it generates power for Southern California. A small café squats above Saddlebag Lake's shoreline, providing simple meals three times a day, small boat rentals, and a water taxi service across the lake. From the campground it's a five-minute walk to the lake for daylong fishing and hiking adventures. Rainbow trout are stocked, but the lake also holds brook, brown, and golden trout.

The elevation here is more than 10,000 feet, and until you adjust, hiking can be a lung-busting experience. A trail departs from the day-use parking lot, heading around the east side of Saddlebag Lake, a less than 4-mile, nearly level hike. The east leg starts out above the lake bisecting a sloping hillside, where you might see Indian paintbrush and yellow wallflower blooming in summer. Small waterfalls gush downhill into the lake, where even from the trail we could see fish swimming in the clear, sapphire blue water. The trail gradually passes through a pocket of pines, then approaches the far end of the lake. Here you can extend the 4-mile experience to an 8-mile hike past a series of spectacular alpine lakes. The trail can be hard to follow near Helen and Shamrock lakes, but there is little elevation change to contend with. Back on the west side of Saddlebag Lake, the trail crosses streams and then slips across a talus slope of rocks shed from the mountain on the right. The journey ends near the dam; continue downhill across the creek to the road, then walk back to the left, and up the campground road (the worst hill of the day). If you are really feeling the elevation or don't care to hike at all, take the water taxi ($9 round-trip) from the boat launch near the café. The taxi makes exploration of the beautiful lakes basin easy.

The café sells firewood but not groceries. If you need ice or other supplies, Lee Vining, 12 miles east

MAP

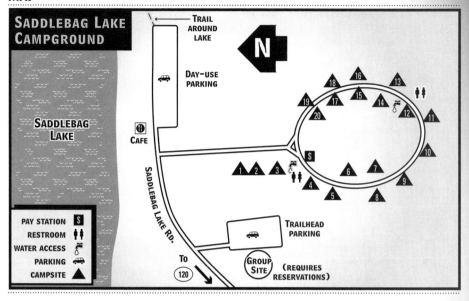

along Interstate 395, has a few small stores, restaurants, and gas. Arriving from the west, the best bet for gas and groceries is the central valley town of Oakdale. Once you begin the climb into Yosemite, there are few places to buy food, and gas prices seem to rise with the elevation. Gas is available year-round at Crane Flat and (until early October at) Tuolumne Meadows, but you'll pay a premium. You can also eat in the restaurant at the Tioga Pass Resort (on the north side of CA 120 just west of Saddlebag Lake Road), and buy ice and limited other supplies there.

The campground at Saddlebag Lake has food-storage lockers. Use them! At 11:30 p.m. a bear walked past our tent, then overturned a cooler in the adjacent campsite. The big bear was run off, but returned at 4 a.m. and ransacked another campsite. We lay in our tent listening to the mayhem. The camp host advises that air horns are particularly effective aids to chase off marauding bears, but the idea of an air horn blast punctuating the quiet of a campground in the middle of the night is less than appealing. For the sake of your fellow campers (and the local bears), keep your food secured in the bear box.

GETTING THERE

From I-5 in San Joaquin County, exit onto CA 120. Drive east through Yosemite. Pass the Tioga Pass entrance station and turn left onto Saddlebag Lake Road. Drive north 2 miles, turn right into the campground. From I-395 in Mono County, turn west on CA 120 for 11 miles, go right onto Saddlebag Lake Road. Drive north 2 miles, and turn right into the campground.

GPS COORDINATES

UTM Zone (WGS84) 11S

Easting 300405

Northing 4204239

Latitude N 37° 57' 50"

Longtitude W 119° 16' 20"

38
TILLIE CREEK CAMPGROUND

> *Tillie Creek is child-friendly and perfect for all seasons.*

TILLIE CREEK IS A CAMPGROUND for all seasons. I love Tillie in the fall when the leaves change; in the winter and spring when it's warm on the plateau and there's snow up above in the mountains that ring the lake; and in the summer when it's hotter than Hades, and all you can do is sit by the water with a beer and a fishing pole.

I also love camping at Tillie Creek with my young niece, because Tillie Creek is very friendly to children. There's a beautiful stream running through the camp that's never fast or deep enough to carry off a child. The lake has a gradually sloping shore. The roads through the campground are just right for young cyclists. There are flushing toilets and hot showers.

This is not the forest primeval. Tillie Creek is what a scout camp or small-town park used to be 30 years ago. There are child-friendly activities in the area, and Wofford Heights is just around the corner for a quick ice cream or a fast-food run.

Look out over Isabella Lake and see the watery grave of ancient Native American villages, historic towns, ranches, and farms—all now submerged. When the dam was built in 1953, water filled the Kern River Valley. When the lake is low, look for a series of snags to find the former courses of the north and south forks of the Kern.

As you drive toward present-day Kernville, note the old cemetery to the right. Around the cemetery sit the foundations of old Kernville. When Isabella Lake was created, the government helped relocate the town to its present site. To get a free map of old Kernville, visit the Kern Valley Museum in Kernville.

In Wofford, head east on Evans Road to visit a site of infamy. Park near the El Segundo Rod and Gun Club and climb the hill just to the south, called the Hill

RATINGS

Beauty: ✿ ✿ ✿ ✿ ✿
Privacy: ✿ ✿ ✿
Spaciousness: ✿ ✿ ✿ ✿
Quiet: ✿ ✿ ✿ ✿
Security: ✿ ✿ ✿
Cleanliness: ✿ ✿ ✿ ✿

of Three Crosses. Look for mortars in the rock where once Tubatulabal Native Americans ground acorns. Here in 1863, Captain Moses McLaughlin and his men massacred a group of Native Americans. At the time, many felt the violence was justified. This can be the basis for a good civics lesson.

To find another historic landmark, drive south on CA 155 to the Keyesville Road. Turn right (southwest) and drive to the end of the paved road. Turn right toward Fort Hill to find all that remains of Keyesville. In 1850, Dickie Keyes, a Cherokee, hit gold-bearing quartz a few hundred yards northwest up Hogeye Gulch. To the south, the Mammoth Mine was found soon afterward and the wild town was born. One of the local hunters who supplied the miners with fresh meat was named Grizzly Adams, because he had two pet grizzly bears. (Remember the TV show of the same name?) Keyesville is long gone, save one house. Built in 1880, it was the scene of a big gunfight involving the "shootin' Walkers." Today, it is occupied and cared for by some locals.

Another interesting trip is to the South Fork Wildlife Area. Go into Kernville and head south on Sierra Way to the wildlife area around South Fork Kern River. Take field glasses and look for the great blue herons that nest in the crowns of trees. Open-minded herons often share trees with owls or hawks. South of the wildlife area are cottonwood and willow stands managed by the Nature Conservancy. The endangered yellow-billed cuckoo and the southwestern willow flycatcher supposedly nest here—I searched for an hour without luck. Apparently, the cuckoos like to eat hairy caterpillars, and the flycatchers fly so fast they are hard to see.

Marinas in the area rent boats, allowing for fun excursions. Remember to bring hats, sunscreen, food, and water. Remember, too, that shallow lakes are more prone to dangerous windblown waves than deep lakes. That has to do with the relationship between waves and the lake bottom (similarly, ocean waves grow taller as they approach the shallows near land).

How can you be in this area and not go river rafting? The trick is to marry the rafting experience

KEY INFORMATION

ADDRESS:	Tillie Creek Campground Sequoia National Forest Greenhorn District P.O. Box 3810 Lake Isabella, CA 92340
OPERATED BY:	Sequoia National Forest
INFORMATION:	(559) 784-1500; www .fs.fed.us/r5/sequoia
OPEN:	Year-round
SITES:	159
EACH SITE HAS:	Picnic table, fire ring
ASSIGNMENT:	First come, first served; reservations recommended
REGISTRATION:	Host will collect on rounds; reserve by phone, (877) 444-6777, or online, www.recreation.gov.
FACILITIES:	Water, flush toilets, hot showers, sanitary disposal station, playground, fish-cleaning station, RV dump station
PARKING:	At site
FEE:	$19–$21, plus $1.50 reservation fee
ELEVATION:	2,650 feet
RESTRICTIONS:	*Pets:* On 6-foot or shorter leash only *Fires:* In fire ring *Alcohol:* No restrictions *Vehicles:* RVs up to 30 feet

MAP

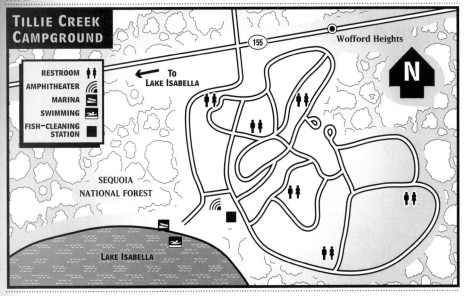

TILLIE CREEK CAMPGROUND

RESTROOM	🚻
AMPHITHEATER	🎦
MARINA	🚤
SWIMMING	🏊
FISH-CLEANING STATION	⬛

← To LAKE ISABELLA

155

Wofford Heights

N

SEQUOIA NATIONAL FOREST

LAKE ISABELLA

GETTING THERE

From L.A., take I-5 north over the Tejon Pass to CA 99. Drive north on CA 99 past Bakersfield. Take CA 178 east to Lake Isabella. Take CA 155 toward Wofford Heights on the west shore of Isabella Lake. The entrance to Tillie Creek Campground is 1 mile before Wofford Heights on the right.

GPS COORDINATES

UTM Zone (WGS84) 11S
Easting 368331
Northing 3951804
Latitude N 35° 42' 05"
Longtitude W 118° 27' 19"

with the age and daring of yourself and your companions. I've been on sedate and bucolic rafting trips and others that turned my hair white. Ask around to find an established rafting company with a solid reputation.

You'll have the most fun, however, just hanging around Tillie Creek Campground. The atmosphere encourages relaxation. The playground attracts and engages children. The changing sun and breeze off the lake combine for an incredible show. Tillie is a place to bring children for a weekend and actually relax.

TRAPPER SPRINGS CAMPGROUND IS CLEAN, uncrowded, and beautiful at a subalpine 8,200 feet. It's a land of granite peaks towering thousands of feet above thick pines, of twisted tamarack and juniper growing out of rock. Courtright Reservoir is a sparkling blue gem against the gray granite, brown tree trunks, and green pine boughs.

What an incredibly beautiful place! John Muir, Scottish sheepherder turned naturalist, wrote:

The Sierra should be called not the Nevada or Snowy Range, but the range of light. And after ten years spent in the heart of it, rejoicing and wondering, bathing in the glorious floods of light, seeing the sunbursts of morning among the icy peaks, the noonday radiance on the trees and rocks and snow, the flush of the alpenglow, and a thousand dashing waterfalls with their marvelous abundance of irised spray, it still seems to me above all others the Range of Light, the most divinely beautiful of all the mountain chains I have ever seen.

Range of Light. That thought stayed with me for the two days my wife and I spent at Trapper Springs. On the first, we walked down the trail to Courtright Reservoir, hiked across the pined granite escarpments at dusk, and drank sundowners on a rock scoured clean by ice, sun, and wind.

The next day, September 15, hunting season began. I expected campgrounds full of gun-toting, beer-swigging NRA-ers and fusillades of rifle fire at dawn. Au contraire, the Trapper Springs Campground attracted just a few polite, gentlemen hunters, and there were a few far-off rifle pops, but otherwise nothing disturbed the sylvan peace of the reservoir and mountainside.

I'm not sure if this state of serenity had anything to do with Marv, our camp host, and his dog, but it's a possibility. The first night, the campground hostess

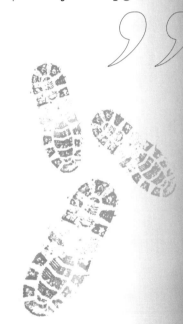

Trapper Springs Campground is an easy-to-access, remote, beautiful campground.

RATINGS

Beauty: ✿ ✿ ✿ ✿ ✿
Privacy: ✿ ✿ ✿ ✿ ✿
Spaciousness: ✿ ✿ ✿ ✿ ✿
Quiet: ✿ ✿ ✿ ✿ ✿
Security: ✿ ✿ ✿ ✿ ✿
Cleanliness: ✿ ✿ ✿ ✿ ✿

KEY INFORMATION

ADDRESS:	Trapper Springs Campground Sierra National Forest High Sierra Ranger District P.O. Box 559 Prather, CA 93651
OPERATED BY:	Pacific Gas & Electric
INFORMATION:	(559) 297-0706; www .fs.fed.us/r5/sierra
OPEN:	May–October
SITES:	75
EACH SITE HAS:	Picnic table, fireplace
ASSIGNMENT:	First come, first served; no reservations
REGISTRATION:	At entrance
FACILITIES:	Water, vault toilets
PARKING:	At site; $3 for additional vehicles
FEE:	$10
ELEVATION:	8,300 feet
RESTRICTIONS:	*Pets:* On leash only; $1 per night *Fires:* In fireplace *Alcohol:* No restrictions *Vehicles:* RVs up to 22 feet *Other:* This is bear country—store food properly; 14-day stay limit.

came by in her golf cart, and we asked her about the hunters. She said, "Well, if they get rowdy, I send my husband Marv down to talk to them, and he takes his dog." Well, we met Marv. He looked rawhide tough, like an ex–rodeo rider, and his dog made your average pit bull look like a French poodle.

The campground was built and is run by Pacific Gas and Electric. They do a fine job. All the facilities are well maintained. The sites are all secluded and clean, and the pitches are well off the service road. The pit toilets are clean. We paid for two sites—9 and 10—sheltered under a huge granite tor.

The campground is located well off the reservoir shore, which keeps the place relatively uncrowded. In Southern California, wherever there's water, there are people. They come for fishing, boating, swimming, and the beauty and primitive peace of mind that a stream or lake provides. So, pick a campground like Trapper Springs that's a little off the water and you won't have too many neighbors.

The trail to the reservoir leaves from the bottom of the second campground loop. The shore is about a quarter of a mile downhill. Or, you can just head north up across the granite escarpments and work your way down. A fishing trail encircles the entire reservoir. There are great places to picnic, sunbathe, and fish. If you fish, be sure to obtain a license and to wear it visibly.

Considering how remote Trapper Springs Campground feels, the road in is pretty mild. Dinkey Creek Road is wide and well graded; you'll thank God for this when you meet the heavily loaded lumber trucks. You'll pass the Ranger Station and small grocery store at Dinkey and head east on McKinley Grove Road. Past the turnoff to Courtright Reservoir Road is the small Wishon Village store and private campground, where you can buy last-minute supplies, including campfire wood. The sign on the door of their saloon reads, "Monday Night Football—Bring your own finger food." Then, head up the hill to Courtright Reservoir; the ascent is gradual, beautiful, and well graded. Before you know it, you're there.

MAP

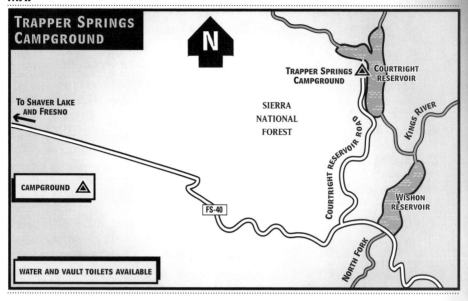

GETTING THERE

From L.A., take I-5 north over the Tejon Pass to CA 99. Drive north on CA 99 past Bakersfield 104 miles to Fresno. Take CA 41 north to CA 168 and go northeast to Shaver Lake. From the town of Shaver Lake, turn east on Dinkey Creek Road and drive 12 miles to McKinley Grove Road. Drive 14 miles to Courtright Reservoir Road. Go left and proceed 12 miles up Courtright Reservoir Road to Trapper Springs Campground.

GPS COORDINATES

UTM Zone (WGS84) 11S
Easting   323628
Northing 4107837
Latitude N 37° 06' 01"
Longtitude W 118° 59' 05"

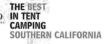

40
TRUMBULL LAKE
CAMPGROUND

> *Don't mind the campground itself. You come for the lakes, the mountains, and the big sky.*

SET DOWN BY THREE TINY jade lakes on the backside of Yosemite, Trumbull Lake Campground is getting popular. It is primitive (no showers), but most of the campsites are reservable. People come back every year. The store in the nearby Virginia Lakes Resort sells beer, ice, and basic supplies. The access road is paved and straight. The fishing is good, the hiking superb. Views of the snowy mountains rising around the three lakes take your breath away. Everybody you meet is complicit, because they are in on the secret that this is the most beautiful spot on Earth.

The campground is on a slope above Trumbull Lake. The tiny lake by the Virginia Lakes Resort is over the hill, and the third lake is just a few hundred yards up the gravel road. The campground is like a scruffy dog. You don't like the way it looks, but after a while you learn to love it. The sites are not well engineered. Many are set too close together or too close to the pit toilets—especially the sites down by the lake. You get the feeling the campground evolved haphazardly, but, hey, here you are, on the far side of nowhere, pretty close to God.

The drive in is spectacular. Come from Los Angeles, and drive up US 395 through the Mojave Desert, the Owens Valley, and up past Mammoth and Mono Lakes. This is the most spectacularly diverse terrain in California, with tons of stuff to do on the way. You can also head up from Los Angeles along the west side of the Sierras, and come across on CA 120 through Yosemite National Parks.

From San Francisco, take CA 108 over the Sonora Pass, where the granite meets the clouds at 9,626 feet. This was the old Sonora and Mono Toll Road, and the men who cut the road had sangfroid. Make sure your

RATINGS

Beauty: ✿ ✿ ✿ ✿ ✿
Privacy: ✿ ✿
Spaciousness: ✿ ✿ ✿
Quiet: ✿ ✿ ✿ ✿ ✿
Security: ✿ ✿ ✿ ✿ ✿
Cleanliness: ✿ ✿ ✿ ✿

flivver is in good shape, and hang on to the steering wheel. It is wild and beautiful—*For Whom the Bell Tolls,* starring Gary Cooper, was filmed here.

I bought salmon eggs and power bait in Lee Vining and caught a decent-sized trout on hooks trimmed of the barb so that I could release (since Tuesday is always spaghetti night). My older sister came along—her first time in the Sierra Nevada for 40 years—and we sat out in the meadow among the lupine and forget-me-nots with a star map and looked up at the sky.

The next day we hiked up to the trailhead by Blue Lake (there's a trail from the campground from Site 5 that connects with the trail past the trailhead) and hiked a mile up to Frog Lakes. This is up around 10,000 feet, so expect to suck some air. Take your time and rest often—the older you get, the longer it takes to get acclimated to the rarer air. Then we plugged on to Summit Lake on the Sierra Ridge between Camiaca Peak and Excelsior Mountain to the south. We stopped for sandwiches and soda chilled in the cold lake water, and watched storm clouds close in around Excelsior Mountain (elevation 12,446 feet). We scooted back down to the campground just ahead of a completely unseasonable (early July) thundershower, replete with ear-cracking thunder, hearty gusts of wind, and frightening, white streaks of lightning.

Cringing in our tent under the pines, I regaled my sister with tales of old John Muir, who loved storms and climbed to the top of the highest pine and tied himself in while the elements raged around him, and shouted Walt Whitmanesque exaltations to the primal gods. And John didn't come back to his tent and a towel; he camped in an old overcoat with his sundries in the pockets. He survived one bone-numbing night by crawling into a hot mud spring—alternating cooking one side of himself and freezing the other.

The next morning the sky was as clear blue as the sea, and the chirping sparrows flitted from bush to flower in the meadow. We borrowed an inflatable boat from a camping neighbor and floated around the lake, trailing a little bait and staring up at the mountains above the basin.

KEY INFORMATION

ADDRESS:	Trumbull Lake Campground Humboldt-Toiyabe National Forest Bridgeport Ranger District HCR 1 Box 1000 Bridgeport, CA 93517
OPERATED BY:	U.S. Forest Service
INFORMATION:	(775) 331-6444; www .fs.fed.us/r4/htnf
OPEN:	Mid-June–mid-October (weather permitting)
SITES:	45 sites for tents or RVs
EACH SITE HAS:	Picnic table, fire ring
ASSIGNMENT:	Some sites offer reservations; others are first come, first served.
REGISTRATION:	At entrance; reserve by phone, (877) 444-6777, or online, www .recreation.gov.
FACILITIES:	Water, vault toilets
PARKING:	At individual sites
FEE:	$15, plus $1.50 reservation fee
ELEVATION:	9,500 feet
RESTRICTIONS:	*Pets:* On leash only *Fires:* In fire ring *Alcohol:* No restrictions *Vehicles:* RVs up to 35 feet *Other:* Don't leave food out, no swimming in lake.

MAP

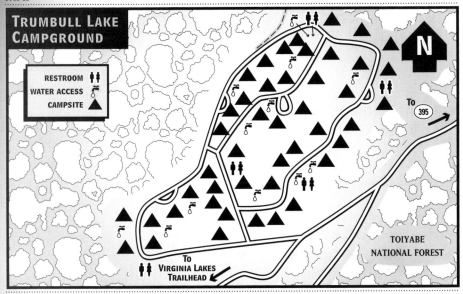

TRUMBULL LAKE CAMPGROUND

RESTROOM	
WATER ACCESS	
CAMPSITE	

To 395

TOIYABE NATIONAL FOREST

To VIRGINIA LAKES TRAILHEAD

GETTING THERE

From Bridgeport, go 14 miles south on US 395 to the Conway Summit. Go right on Virginia Lakes Road, drive 6 miles to the campground on the right. From Lee Vining, drive 12 miles north on US 395 to the Conway Summit and go left on Virginia Lakes Road. Drive 6 miles to the campground on the right.

I spoke to the campground host (from L & L Inc.), who told me they had plans to make more of the campsites reservable. I checked out all the sites. Sites 10 through 13 are lakeside with a great view, but there's heavy traffic and they're near a pit toilet. I preferred the campsites off the lake, around the fringes of the camp. Site 4 was my favorite. After that came sites 5, 7, 8 (not Site 6), and 35 through 37. Still, the campsite itself doesn't really matter. Shortly after arriving at Trumbull Lake Campground, as soon as you take a good look around at the mountains and water, you'll know you're home.

GPS COORDINATES

UTM Zone (WGS84) 11S
Easting 301898
Northing 4212836
Latitude N 38° 03' 02"
Longtitude W 119° 15' 28"

THE TWIN LAKES AROUND THE Twin Lakes Campground look like blue beans joined at the hip. A little bridge connects the two lakes, and folks in rental rowboats and canoes scoot underneath it. Grandfathers teach their grandchildren how to fish as a waterfall cascades down the cliff above the lakes.

The campground is both accessible and friendly. There are rustic cabins, a lodge, and a store. A few miles away, in the city of Mammoth Lakes, you'll find pizzerias, hardware stores, and a big, wonderful Vons Supermarket on Old Mammoth Road. Twin Lakes Campground is a great place to camp for a week; bring your family for the summer vacation.

The campsites sprawl around the two lakes and uphill across the road. If you find Twin Lakes Campground full, head a few hundred yards up the road to beautiful Coldwater Campground on Coldwater Creek. Or, head a mile or so up to Lake Mary Campground and Lake George Campground. All the sites are wonderful, but none is reservable. Phone the rangers to check on site availability and plan your trip so you arrive either in off-season or by Thursday for the weekend.

Head to the top of Coldwater Campground and walk a few hundred yards to the old Mammoth Consolidated Gold Mine on Mineral Hill. Here, you can see some of the old buildings from the mining towns and locations of the many bawdy houses and a saloon named The Temple of Folly (long-since destroyed). Walk around the old buildings and rusted machinery and imagine the men who sweated in the summer sun and froze in the winter, obsessed with gold. Climb up to the upper adit in the early morning for a view of Mount Banner and Mount Ritter.

Take the nice little hike to Emerald Lake. It's about

> *A perfect place to spend summer vacation with the family.*

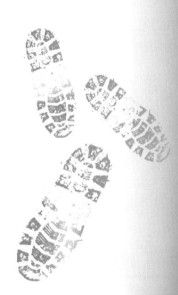

RATINGS

Beauty: ✿ ✿ ✿ ✿ ✿
Privacy: ✿ ✿ ✿ ✿
Spaciousness: ✿ ✿ ✿ ✿ ✿
Quiet: ✿ ✿ ✿
Security: ✿ ✿ ✿ ✿ ✿
Cleanliness: ✿ ✿ ✿ ✿ ✿

KEY INFORMATION

ADDRESS: Twin Lakes Campground Mammoth Ranger Station 2500 Main Street Mammoth Lakes, CA 93546

OPERATED BY: U.S. Forest Service

INFORMATION: (760) 873-2400; www.fs.fed.us/r5/inyo

OPEN: May 25–October 31

SITES: 95

EACH SITE HAS: Picnic table, fireplace

ASSIGNMENT: First come, first served; no reservations

REGISTRATION: At entrance, reserve by phone (877) 444-6777, or online, www.recreation.gov.

FACILITIES: Water, flush toilets, boat rental, wheelchair-accessible sites

PARKING: At site

FEE: $19

ELEVATION: 8,700 feet

RESTRICTIONS: *Pets:* On leash only
Fires: In fireplaces
Alcohol: No restrictions
Vehicles: RVs up to 22 feet
Other: To reduce vehicle traffic into Devil's Postpile, a shuttle bus system has been implemented. Campers pay a one-time fee exemption. Stop at the Mammoth Lakes visitor center (on the way into Mammoth Lakes) or the Adventure Center (at the ski area) for more information.

a mile up the mountain. The trailhead and parking lot are next to the parking lot for the mine on Mineral Hill. Walk up by Coldwater Creek where there are lupine, monkey flower, and fireweed. Bring a picnic and climb the rocks around the lake. Bring fishing gear as well. I watched one older woman reel in two decent trout while I ate my sandwich.

If you are ambitious, go around the left side of Emerald Lake. At the signed junction, go right to Gentian Meadow–Sky Meadows. Climb up by the inlet creek and reach tiny Gentian Meadow. Carry on up past a waterfall, and then, after a while, you'll reach Sky Meadows. Look for paintbrush, corn lily, and elephant's heads among the grass. It's about 2.5 miles back down the hill.

Or, if you are truly ambitious, pick up the trail to Duck Pass (8.2 miles round-trip) back in the parking lot by the trailhead to Emerald Lake. Find the Duck Pass sign and start climbing. When you reach the entry sign for the John Muir Wilderness, bear right. Climb up through lodgepoles, pines, and hemlocks, and carry on past the trail to Arrowhead Lake, Skelton Lake, and Barney Lake. Next, you'll see alpine Duck Pass ahead, with all the high elevation flowers—columbine, gentian, and sorrel. Finally, traverse the pass and you'll see Duck Lake and pretty little Pika Lake on the left.

Back at Twin Lakes Campground, a nice stroll is around the shore to the falls. Access the trail behind Campsite 24. You'll see a sign that says "Private Road." Bear left and follow the trail that heads through the trees to the waterfall. Or, walk over to Tamarack Lodge. This graceful establishment was built in 1923. The clerk from the grocery store averred that Tamarack Lodge has the best food in Mammoth Lakes.

However, my wife and I ate chez campsite the last time I was at Twin Lakes. I boiled some quartered potatoes and set them aside. Then I fried some onions, garlic, jalapeño peppers, and strips of chicken breast in the pot. After a bit, I returned the potatoes to the pot and stirred it all about. Very delicious for a one-pot meal!

About 3:15 a.m., I heard a visitor. I jumped out of my sleeping bag and poked my head out of the tent. A

MAP

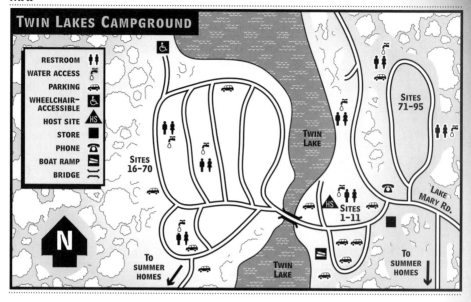

TWIN LAKES CAMPGROUND

RESTROOM
WATER ACCESS
PARKING
WHEELCHAIR-ACCESSIBLE
HOST SITE
STORE
PHONE
BOAT RAMP
BRIDGE

SITES 16–70

SITES 1–11

SITES 71–95

TWIN LAKE

LAKE MARY RD.

To SUMMER HOMES

TWIN LAKE

To SUMMER HOMES

N

three-foot bear was rifling through my cooler of soft drinks. I shouted, and the midget bear looked at me insolently and pawed on. I threw a pebble, and he ran over to a tree and climbed up a few feet. I retrieved my cooler. He gave me the evil eye and ran into the underbrush. The next morning he was rooting around in the big trash container down by the bridge. He glared at me and sauntered off, combing garbage out of his whiskers.

GETTING THERE

From L.A., take I-5 north to CA 14. Go north to US 395 near Inyokern. Go north on US 395 for 123 miles to Bishop. Continue 37 miles north on US 395 to Mammoth Lakes. From Mammoth Lakes, go west 3 miles on Lake Mary Road to the campground.

GPS COORDINATES

UTM Zone (WGS84) 11S
Easting 294151
Northing 4225387
Latitude N 38° 09' 10"
Longtitude W 119° 20' 58"

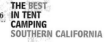

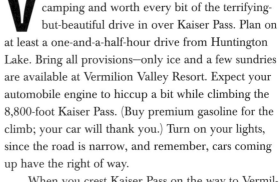

> *Vermilion Campground proves that the best and most beautiful camping is usually the least accessible.*

VERMILION **CAMPGROUND IS SUPERB** tent camping and worth every bit of the terrifying-but-beautiful drive in over Kaiser Pass. Plan on at least a one-and-a-half-hour drive from Huntington Lake. Bring all provisions—only ice and a few sundries are available at Vermilion Valley Resort. Expect your automobile engine to hiccup a bit while climbing the 8,800-foot Kaiser Pass. (Buy premium gasoline for the climb; your car will thank you.) Turn on your lights, since the road is narrow, and remember, cars coming up have the right of way.

When you crest Kaiser Pass on the way to Vermillion, look out over the San Joaquin River Canyon and Kaiser Wilderness. John Muir wrote: "Westward, the general flank of the range is seen flowing sublimely away from the sharp summits, in smooth undulations; a sea of huge gray granite waves dotted with lakes and meadows, and fluted with stupendous canyons that grow steadily deeper as they recede into the distance."

At Vermillion, most sites are for tents only. This is no easy access for RVs, and most of the parking places are too short or steep for RVs. The pitches and picnic tables are a respectable distance away as well. At the campground you'll find sandy beaches and granite, pined points creating private coves and bays.

The swimming in Lake Edison was great. Granted, I was there in September, but you don't have to be a polar bear to enjoy jumping in and splashing around. Bring little rubber shoes for the children, so they can race through the shallows.

A friendly couple camping near my wife and me invited us to use their kayaks. We paddled east for about a half mile and beached on an island about 300 yards offshore. I swam and then lay on hot granite slabs and looked across at the snow fields on the

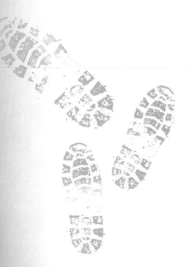

RATINGS

Beauty: ✿ ✿ ✿ ✿ ✿
Privacy: ✿ ✿ ✿ ✿ ✿
Spaciousness: ✿ ✿ ✿ ✿
Quiet: ✿ ✿ ✿ ✿
Security: ✿ ✿ ✿ ✿ ✿
Cleanliness: ✿ ✿ ✿ ✿ ✿

mountains ringing the canyon. On a boat trolling by, I saw a guy pull in at least a three-pound trout. What an incredible place!

The Vermilion Valley Resort runs a water ferry, which leaves the resort at 9:30 a.m. It drops you off to the east at the head of the lake, where the fishing is spectacular. Some folks hike up the trail toward Mono Pass, and some just lie around and wait for the ferry to come pick them up at 4 p.m. The round-trip costs $15, and you can bring your dog for free.

You can also hike east of the campground about a mile to a respectable brook. There is a bridge about 300 yards north, or you can wade across and freeze your feet off. This water comes off a glacier for sure. A little farther, the trail splits. The left fork heads up Silver Pass to the John Muir Trail/Pacific Crest Trail. The right fork takes you 15 miles up to Mono Pass and down the other side to Rock Creek below Mammoth (using the ferry cuts miles off this hike).

The resort rents boats for about $50 a day. This is reasonable, especially when you consider the alternative of trailering a boat up over Kaiser Pass. The resort also has a little café and rents some basic rooms. You can take a classy hot-spring soak in a deep tub at Mono Hot Springs.

Try to pick a campsite at Vermilion well away from the resort, since they run a generator until about 10 p.m. Wood is at a premium, and bundles are expensive at the resort store. Instead, bring a saw. East of the camp, along the trail to the brook, there are quite a few deadfalls. The sand around the pitches is fine and invasive. It's a good idea to bring along a bucket to dip your feet in before entering your tent. Bring a small brush to clean out the tent floor.

Be sure to check with rangers about the water before you arrive. The water at Vermilion is wonderful and spills out of a 400-foot artesian well, but, the day we left, an inspector came through and posted the water spigots with "not safe to drink" signs. I wished I'd brought a filter to purify the lake water, because the only other alternative was boiling it. Luckily, an hour later, the water scare turned out to be a false alarm.

KEY INFORMATION

ADDRESS:	Vermilion Campground Sierra National Forest High Sierra Ranger District P.O. Box 559 Prather, CA 93651
OPERATED BY:	Sierra National Forest
INFORMATION:	(559) 297-0706; www .fs.fed.us/r5/sierra
OPEN:	June–September
SITES:	11 tent sites, 20 sites for tents or RVs
EACH SITE HAS:	Picnic table, fireplace
ASSIGNMENT:	First come, first served; reservations recommended
REGISTRATION:	At entrance; reserve by phone, (877) 444-6777, or online, www.recreation.gov.
FACILITIES:	Water, vault toilets
PARKING:	At or near site
FEE:	$17, plus $1.50 reservation fee
ELEVATION:	7,000 feet
RESTRICTIONS:	*Pets:* On leash only *Fires:* In fireplace *Alcohol:* No restrictions *Vehicles:* RVs up to 16 feet *Other:* 15-mph limit for boats on Lake Edison; 14-day stay limit

MAP

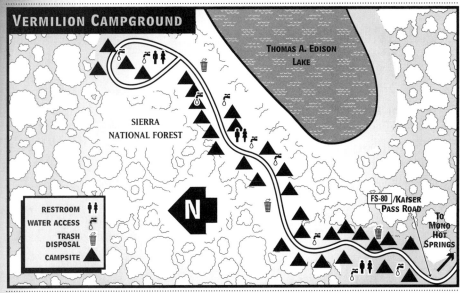

VERMILION CAMPGROUND

THOMAS A. EDISON LAKE

SIERRA NATIONAL FOREST

FS-80 /KAISER PASS ROAD

TO MONO HOT SPRINGS

RESTROOM
WATER ACCESS
TRASH DISPOSAL
CAMPSITE

GETTING THERE

From L.A., take I-5 north over the Tejon Pass to CA 99. Drive north on CA 99 past Bakersfield 104 miles to Fresno. Take CA 41 north to CA 168. Go northeast (right) to Shaver Lake. From Shaver Lake, head 20 miles north on CA 168 to Huntington Lake. From Lake Shore on Huntington Lake, take Kaiser Pass Road (FS 80) to Edison Lake Road at Mono Hot Springs. Continue 5 miles north to Vermilion Campground.

If Vermilion is full, head back down the road a few miles to Mono Creek Campground. Or, try Mono Hot Springs, which has 26 sites. Because there is no dispersed camping in the area, the only other alternative is Jackass Meadow below the Florence Lake dam.

GPS COORDINATES

UTM Zone (WGS84) 11S
Easting 321983
Northing 4138814
Latitude N 37° 22' 44"
Longtitude W 119° 00' 38"

YOSEMITE NATIONAL PARK IS HEAVEN on earth. With the Mariposa Battalion, the first English-speaking party to see Yosemite Valley, was Lafayette Bunnell. He wrote: "The grandeur of the scene was softened by the haze that hung over the valley—light as gossamer—and by the clouds which partially dimmed the higher cliffs and mountains. This obscurity of vision merely increased the awe with which I beheld it, and as I looked, a peculiar exalted sensation seemed to fill my whole being, and I found my eyes in tears with emotion."

The Yosemite Native Americans, the original inhabitants, loved the valley too, but the arrival of the forty-niners ended their resiliency. By 1852, Chief Tenaya of the Yosemites, his tribe decimated, was stoned to death by some raiding Mono Native Americans. Soon after, August T. Dowd, a miner hunting in the valley, saw a tree bigger than he'd ever seen before. He told his friends about it, and the tourists began flooding in. Yosemite Valley became a mecca to the world.

Now, four-hour traffic jams in Yosemite Valley are common, and the campgrounds are constantly booked. Avoid Yosemite Valley, and explore the rest of the park instead. Come in from the east over the Tioga Pass off US 395 or from the west on CA 120. Shun CA 41, and don't get stuck in the Wawona Tunnel.

However, you should see Tuolumne Meadows and camp in White Wolf Campground. John Muir eloquently described the Tioga Pass area: "From garden to garden, ridge to ridge, I drifted enchanted, now on my knees gazing into the face of a daisy, now climbing again and again among the purple and azure flowers of the hemlocks, now down into the treasuries of the snow, or gazing far over domes and peaks, lakes and woods, and the billowy glaciated fields of the upper

> *White Wolf Campground is the only campground in Yosemite National Park worth squeezing into.*

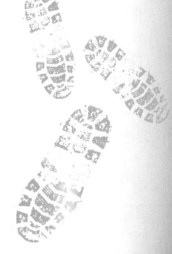

RATINGS

Beauty: ✮ ✮ ✮ ✮ ✮
Privacy: ✮ ✮ ✮ ✮ ✮
Spaciousness: ✮ ✮ ✮ ✮ ✮
Quiet: ✮ ✮ ✮ ✮ ✮
Security: ✮ ✮ ✮ ✮ ✮
Cleanliness: ✮ ✮ ✮ ✮ ✮

ADDRESS:	White Wolf Campground Yosemite National Park P.O. Box 577 Yosemite, CA 95389
OPERATED BY:	National Park Service
INFORMATION:	(209) 372-8502; www.nps.gov/yose; for recorded information, call (209) 372-0200.
OPEN:	July–September
SITES:	74
EACH SITE HAS:	Picnic table, fireplace, food-storage cabinet
ASSIGNMENT:	First come, first served; no reservations
REGISTRATION:	At entrance
FACILITIES:	Water, flush toilets, food storage lockers
PARKING:	At site
FEE:	$14; must pay $20 Yosemite National Park entrance fee
ELEVATION:	8,000 feet
RESTRICTIONS:	*Pets:* On leash only *Fires:* In fireplace *Alcohol:* No restrictions *Vehicles:* RVs up to 27 feet *Other:* 14-day stay limit; keep food stored properly from bears.

Tuolumne. In the midst of such beauty, pierced with its rays, one's body is all one tingling palate. Who wouldn't be a mountaineer! Up here all the world's prizes seem nothing."

White Wolf Campground is full of tiny meadows and stands of lodgepole pine, and the Middle Tuolumne River flows through the campground. The sites are set among the pines and granite boulders. The campground is constructed beautifully; each loop seems miles away from the others. The arrangement of the tables and sites create a sense of spaciousness. The facilities are clean and well tended. This is slow, elegant camping.

Only the little bear wandering around camp caused a little nervousness. Obviously he was a special bear because he had little colored tags in his ears. Our neighbor shook a towel at the little bear, and he decamped, at least for that day. Of course, we were careful to put away our coolers even if we were only leaving camp for a moment. Bears get a record for raiding campers, and the rangers are forced to take steps. We didn't want that to happen to the little bear with tags in his ears.

We hiked up to Hardin Lake and sat under the pines reading John Muir. Muir cavorted through these mountains, wearing a great coat, and carried all his gear in his pockets. At night, he lay down in the same mas-sive coat and slept. Those old-timers were real men!

Take John A. "Snowshoe" Thompson, for example. Every winter from 1856 to 1876, Thompson carried the U.S. mail alone across the Sierra. Traveling on skis (called snowshoes in those days), Thompson carried a 100-pound pack and made the 180-mile round-trip in five days. His diet consisted of beef jerky and crackers, and he drank snow. He didn't carry a blanket or wear an overcoat.

At night, Thompson would find a tree stump. After setting fire to the stump, he'd cut some fir boughs for a bed. With his feet to the fire, he'd sleep through the worst blizzards. If he was caught outside camp in a bad blizzard, he just stood on a rock and danced a jig to stay warm.

MAP

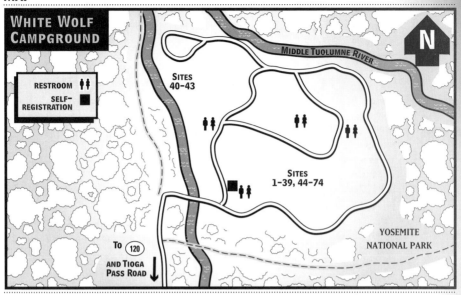

WHITE WOLF CAMPGROUND

RESTROOM

SELF-REGISTRATION

MIDDLE TUOLUMNE RIVER

SITES 40–43

SITES 1–39, 44–74

YOSEMITE NATIONAL PARK

To 120

AND TIOGA PASS ROAD

Today, camping life is a little easier. Still, remember to get supplies in the western flatlands or in Mammoth Lakes on your way in from the east. Only ice, beer, and soda are available in Tuolumne Meadows, Crane Flat, and White Wolf Lodge near White Wolf Campground (in the summer months only).

GETTING THERE

From L.A., take I-5 north to CA 14. Head north to US 395 near Inyokern. Go north on US 395 for 123 miles to Bishop. Continue north on US 395 for 57 miles to CA 120 (Tioga Pass Road). Go west 43 miles to White Wolf Road on the right. The White Wolf Campground is about a mile down that road.

GPS COORDINATES

UTM Zone (WGS84) 11S
Easting 267162
Northing 4194776
Latitude N 37° 52' 15"
Longtitude W 119° 38' 50"

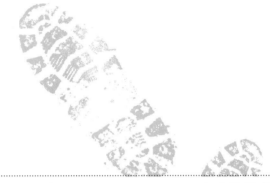

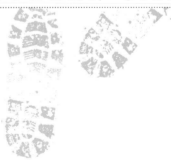

THE SOUTHERN SIERRAS

44
DARK CANYON CAMPGROUND

I DROVE THROUGH IDYLLWILD in a mist so thick the neon lights of the cute little mountain town could only blush through the fog. I found a place to park and drifted along a sidewalk until I ran right into a Mount San Jacinto State Park ranger who said this fog never happens this time of year. It was June 15; it was supposed to be sunny and at least 80°F.

Back on CA 243, I leaned out the window and navigated by the stripes down the middle of the highway until Forest Service Road 4S02 split off to the right, and I could reckon the road by aiming for the gap in the pines. After traveling down the narrowing road and across a stream, I was at Dark Canyon Campground, one of the most charming campgrounds in the very charming Idyllwild area of the San Bernardinos.

Upon arrival, it took me a minimal amount of time to find the perfect campsite down by the stream that runs through the canyon. The water is cold and runs clear around granite boulders through pools with clean sand bottoms. In this area, and most parts of the San Bernardino National Forest, water is at a premium.

The 17 campsites in Dark Canyon are perfect for tent camping. The fireplaces and picnic tables for some of the sites are a 15-yard walk away from the parking lot (ample enough for an RV, however). Five sites are located down by the stream and the rest are up in the pines above the campground.

Shortly after I arrived, it started snowing, and my hike around the canyon was screened through the hard-driving sleet and wet snow. What I saw were pines; Dark Canyon is right on the line between north-facing Upper Chaparral and the higher Yellow Pine Forest. Both of these areas are packed with pines: Coulter pine, white fir, incense cedar, sugar and yellow pine. Down by the stream, you'll see riparian trees like alder, willow, and black cottonwood.

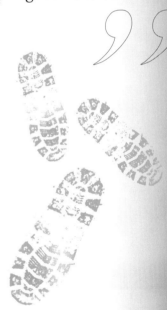

> *Dark Canyon Campground is a heartbreaker so beautiful and so near Los Angeles. Reserve!*

RATINGS

Beauty: ✿ ✿ ✿ ✿ ✿
Privacy: ✿ ✿ ✿ ✿
Spaciousness: ✿ ✿ ✿ ✿
Quiet: ✿ ✿ ✿ ✿ ✿
Security: ✿ ✿ ✿ ✿ ✿
Cleanliness: ✿ ✿ ✿ ✿ ✿

KEY INFORMATION

I hiked a mile or so up the dirt road to the trailhead that heads east into Mount San Jacinto State Park to Deer Springs. By this time, it was sleeting harder, so I endeavored to collect some dry wood and light a fire in my fireplace. Fortunately, I had a can of charcoal lighter fluid, which, when combined with a little dry paper and a modest amount of kindling, will start up just about any campground wood. I know lighter fluid doesn't sound kosher to the former Boy Scout planning a camping trip at home in the living room, but, when everyone is blowing and fanning wet pine needles and wet wood, this petroleum distillate cheater can make you look like a hero. On the other hand, hardware stores also sell a small hatchet-sized splitter, which does a good job chopping wood into more easily lit kindling if you can't handle the humiliation of the tenderfoot charcoal fluid.

Dark Canyon is very popular. The campground hostess told me it usually fills up early Friday afternoon for the weekends. On big weekends, she recommended arriving on Thursday. It's a great idea to make a reservation.

If you decide not to reserve, look for the sign on FS 4S02 informing you if Dark Canyon Campground and its two sister campgrounds, Fern Basin and Marion Mountain, are full. If so, drive to Idyllwild and go to the Ranger Station on the left as you enter town. They will direct you to dispersed camping areas. Some of these are "yellow post" areas, which means you can have a fire in the metal fire ring. Other areas require a fire permit, which will be issued at the station if fire conditions allow it.

Other alternatives include the two Mount San Jacinto State Park campgrounds. Idyllwild Campground is right smack in town by the Mount San Jacinto State Park Ranger Station. It is clean (flush toilets and showers), safe, and especially wonderful on Sunday morning when you feel like walking 100 yards to Idyllwild for brunch and the Sunday paper. Many of Idyllwild's sites are for tents only, which makes the campground especially friendly. Stone Creek is out of town and a little more primitive.

MAP

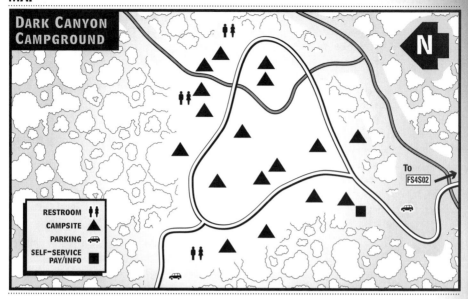

DARK CANYON CAMPGROUND

N

To FS4S02

RESTROOM
CAMPSITE
PARKING
SELF—SERVICE PAY/INFO

The last time I visited, Stone Creek Campground was closed. I asked a particularly crusty ranger why. "Plague," he said. "My God, I guess I don't want to camp there!" I whined. "Oh, hell!" he said. "We're just going to dust all the squirrels down for fleas, and that's that." He'd be damned if he ever heard of anybody getting the plague from squirrels and allowed that it was no reason to give up camping. "Just don't feed the little beggars corn chips and you'll be all right," he assured me.

GETTING THERE

From L.A., drive east on I-10 to Banning. Take CA 243 south 22 miles toward Idyllwild. Turn left on FS 4S02 and go another 3 miles to the campground.

GPS COORDINATES

UTM Zone (WGS84) 11S
Easting 524798
Northing 3740448
Latitude N 33° 48' 14"
Longtitude W 116° 43' 56"

45
DOANE VALLEY CAMPGROUND

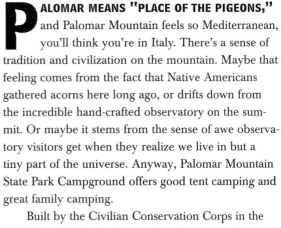

> *See the stars at Palomar Observatory, eat at Mother's Kitchen Restaurant, and bring home ten pounds of gems.*

PALOMAR MEANS "PLACE OF THE PIGEONS," and Palomar Mountain feels so Mediterranean, you'll think you're in Italy. There's a sense of tradition and civilization on the mountain. Maybe that feeling comes from the fact that Native Americans gathered acorns here long ago, or drifts down from the incredible hand-crafted observatory on the summit. Or maybe it stems from the sense of awe observatory visitors get when they realize we live in but a tiny part of the universe. Anyway, Palomar Mountain State Park Campground offers good tent camping and great family camping.

Built by the Civilian Conservation Corps in the 1930s (when folks tent-camped and cars were tiny Fords), the campsites are styled in stone and set under huge trees. The toilets are clean, and the hot showers cost a few quarters. The park headquarters is back up the road on the way in and, when I was there, was staffed by a helpful lady ranger who looked like a young Elke Sommer. Included in the park area is a Christian Conference Center and a School Camp, both infested with boisterous junior-high schoolers. If you tire of camp grub, at the intersection of County Road S6 and S7, you'll find Mother's Kitchen Restaurant, which serves good food.

Near the campground is Doane's Pond, a cute pond with picnic tables set around it under ramadas, because it gets hot here in the summer. On the road in, you'll see a sign threatening a $500 fine for miscreants throwing snowballs at cars or people, so you know snow drifts up a bit here in the winter. I think the best time to visit is in the spring or fall. But, the Palomar Observatory qualifies the mountain as a wonderful place to visit year-round. I think it's easier to view ourselves as creatures of the larger universe when camping than when home watching television. Buy the star

RATINGS

Beauty: ✰ ✰ ✰
Privacy: ✰ ✰ ✰ ✰
Spaciousness: ✰ ✰ ✰
Quiet: ✰ ✰ ✰
Security: ✰ ✰ ✰ ✰ ✰
Cleanliness: ✰ ✰ ✰ ✰

map in the observatory gift shop and go out in the meadow by Doane's Pond at night. Imagine how the ancients must have felt in a world lit only by starlight and fire.

I followed a group of junior-high schoolers and heard their teacher try to pique the loutish pupils' interest in the observatory. It really is amazing. The dome weighs 1,000 tons and is so well engineered that it can be moved by hand. The telescope, which weighs 750 tons, can also be moved by the touch of a finger. The glass disk at the heart of the telescope was ground and polished to the two-millionth part of an inch. Incredible!

It wasn't hard to spot the band-tailed pigeon that gives Palomar Mountain its name. The band-tail is not your ordinary "rat with wings" pigeon cadging food at the local patio restaurant, but a lovely bird with a yellow bill, green nape, and white neck band. Its call is a low-pitched, owl-like "coo-coo."

Like the band-tail, the acorn woodpecker eats acorns. It goes around storing them by the thousands in specially drilled holes—each containing a single acorn—in dead trees, telephone poles, fence posts, and even the sides of buildings. Its diligence is equaled only by the gray squirrel, which hides acorns in underground caches and later smells them out. Acorns are a big industry on the mountain.

The Luiseno Native Americans, who also collected acorns on Palomar, ate manzanita berries, choke cherries, and toyon berries. For salad and veggies, they ate lily bulbs, tree mushrooms, yucca blossoms, sage shoots, wild mustard, clover, and celery. In season, they relished watercress, lamb's quarter, and Indian lettuce. Palomar is a bountiful mountain.

If you don't find a site at Doane Valley Campground (reserve ahead for weekends!), there are two Forest Service camps up the road to the observatory. At wide-open Observatory Campground there are huge oaks and views of the ridges. Just a quarter-mile up is Fry Creek Campground, a nice campground in the woods that favors tent campers because the road in is too narrow for RVs or trailers.

KEY INFORMATION

ADDRESS:	Doane Valley Campground Palomar Mountain State Park 19952 State Park Road Palomar Mountain, CA 92060
OPERATED BY:	California State Parks
INFORMATION:	(760) 742-3462; www.parks.ca.gov; for information on neighboring Cleveland National Forest call (858) 673-6180
OPEN:	Year-round
SITES:	21 for tents only, 10 for RVs
EACH SITE HAS:	Fireplace, picnic table
ASSIGNMENT:	First come, first served; reservations required
REGISTRATION:	At entrance; reserve by phone, (877) 444-6777, or online, www.reserve america.com.
FACILITIES:	Water, flush toilets, coin-operated hot showers, firewood for sale, wheelchair-accessible sites
PARKING:	Near site
FEE:	$20 ($15 off-season)
ELEVATION:	4,700 feet
RESTRICTIONS:	*Pets:* On leash only; not allowed on trails *Fires:* In fireplace; may be prohibited during high fire danger *Alcohol:* No restrictions *Vehicles:* RVs up to 27 feet *Other:* Stay limit of 7 consecutive days; 30 days annually; no off-road travel

MAP

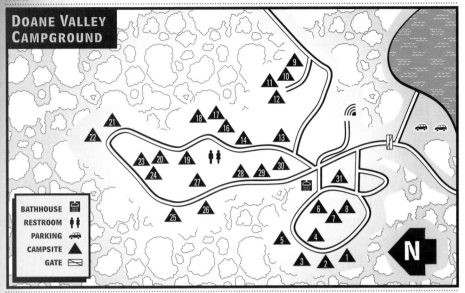

DOANE VALLEY CAMPGROUND

BATHHOUSE
RESTROOM
PARKING
CAMPSITE
GATE

N

GETTING THERE

From L.A., drive east on I-10. Take I-15 south to the intersection with CA 76. Drive east 21 miles to CR S-6. Go north (left) 6.8 miles, then left on CR S-7 3 miles to the campground.

A good side trip from Palomar is to Gems of Pala, just down the road toward I-15. It's open Thursday through Sunday, 10 a.m. to 4 p.m. For a fee, you get to dig in one of the world's foremost tourmaline locations. Bring a garden shovel, a spray bottle, and a one-eighth-inch mesh screen about one foot by two feet. You get to take home up to ten pounds of pink, blue, green, black, and watermelon tourmaline. Call Gems of Pala at (760) 742-1356 for information.

GPS COORDINATES

UTM Zone (WGS84) 11S
Easting 509193
Northing 3683424
Latitude N 33° 20' 38"
Longtitude W 116° 54' 04"

46
HANNA FLAT
CAMPGROUND

"**A**BANDON HOPE ALL YE WHO** enter here" is a good motto for campers coming to Big Bear Lake on holiday weekends, but during mid-week or off-season, the north shore is downright civilized. It's a beautiful place, and the rangers and civilians are genuinely friendly.

Hanna Flat Campground features good tent camping. The sites are set in stands of Jeffrey pine and spaced nicely to allow vistas of pine-covered and rocky hills with the blue-sky, big-country look. Manzanita grows under the pines, and there's a mild riparian community by the cut along the campground. Best of all, the sites are engineered to give campers maximum privacy and space. Each site has an abundance of flat, spongy, and pine-needled ground.

Hanna Flat Campground is run by Alpine Camping Services, a private company, and they do a good job. When we visited Hanna Flat they were represented by a Grizzly Adams–type fellow in rawhide boots, and by his dad back at the Camp Host trailer. There are clean pit and flush toilets.

The few miles of dirt road coming in discourages most RVers, who prefer a site down by the lake in parks with hookups. In the nearby village of Fawnskin, you'll find a little grocery store and two homespun eateries. For serious shopping go around the lake to Big Bear City. There's a Thrifty as big as an aircraft carrier and more banks than you can shake a stick at.

Lake access from Hanna Flat Campground begins in Fawnskin's Dana Point Marina, which has a bait shop, picnic tables, a lake beach, and toilets. A sign announces roosting bald eagles from November to March. Fawnskin is charming. I loved all the rustic wood cottages.

More lake access lies below Serrano Camground, a few miles east of Fawnskin. There's a marina that rents

"Big Sky" country, with fishing, biking, and hiking. But don't get caught alive here on big holidays.

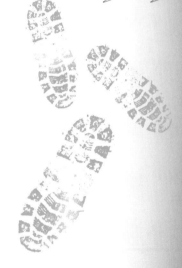

RATINGS

Beauty: ✪ ✪ ✪ ✪
Privacy: ✪ ✪ ✪ ✪ ✪
Spaciousness: ✪ ✪ ✪ ✪ ✪
Quiet: ✪ ✪ ✪ ✪ ✪
Security: ✪ ✪ ✪ ✪ ✪
Cleanliness: ✪ ✪ ✪ ✪ ✪

ADDRESS: Hanna Flat
Campground
San Bernardino
National Forest
Big Bear Discovery
Center
P.O. Box 66
North Shore Drive,
CA 38
Fawnskin, CA 92333

OPERATED BY: California Land
Management

INFORMATION: (909) 382-2790;
www.fs.fed.us/r5/
sanbernardino/
recreation/camping/
index.shtml

OPEN: May 14–October 10

SITES: 88 (43 reservable)

EACH SITE HAS: Picnic table,
fire ring

ASSIGNMENT: Some sites offer
reservations; others
are first come, first
served.

REGISTRATION: At entrance (or with
host); reserve by
phone, (877) 444-
6777, or online,
www.recreation.gov.

FACILITIES: Water, flush toilets,
firewood for sale

PARKING: At site

FEE: $20

ELEVATION: 7,000 feet

RESTRICTIONS: *Pets:* On leash only
Fires: In fire ring
Alcohol: No
restrictions
Vehicles: RVs up to 40
feet; fee for second
vehicle
Other: 14-day stay
limit

boats and bicycles, an observatory, a paved hiking and biking path, and Meadow's Edge Picnic Ground, with all the amenities and a nice lake beach. The observatory dome is out on the water at the end of a dock, because water cuts down on image distortion. Noted for its study of the sun, the observatory is open to the public Saturdays during July and August, from 4 to 6 p.m.

Just past Serrano Campground is the Big Bear Ranger Station, where you can get maps of all the hiking trails. Big Bear offers good hiking and is a world-renowned mountain-biking center. Snow Summit, a snow-ski resort, utilizes its chairlifts in the summer to carry mountain bikers to the top of the mountain, at 8,200 feet, where there are 60 miles of accessible trails. The real fanatics go down Snow Summit's single-track downhills at about 90 miles per hour.

Back at the Hanna Flat Campground, you'll find two fun hikes; one heads out from Site 51 to Grout Bay, and the other goes from Site 25 north and back along the road. The trail to Grout Bay is an 8-mile round-trip with lovely views of the lake from the plateau. Look for eagles on the tops of dead trees. From this trail, you can also access the trail to Gray's Peak. The trail is a bit rough as you near the summit.

The second hike takes you north to the beaver dams on Holcomb Creek. Here, beavers live in dens in caves along the water's edge. To more easily access the dams, drive your car out of the campground, turn left on the dirt road you came in on (FS 3N14), and go a mile or so to a parking lot on the right before Holcomb Creek. Find the Pacific Crest Trail just north across the creek and to the left of FS 3N14. Follow the trail west about a mile to see the beaver dams. Look for wildflowers along the way. I was able to identify wild rose, lupine, Indian paintbrush, and scarlet bugler.

Look at the mountains around Big Bear Lake and imagine—this was once the bottom of the ocean! Of course, that was about 600 million years ago. Then, 60 million years ago, the earth's plates ground together and pushed the ocean floor up to make the San Bernardinos.

The Big Bear Lake area can get crowded, so time your visits for maximum enjoyment. As you drive up

MAP

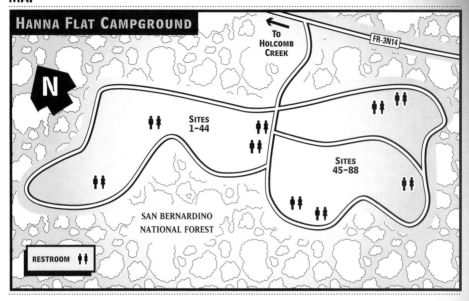

HANNA FLAT CAMPGROUND

To HOLCOMB CREEK

FR-3N14

N

SITES 1-44

SITES 45-88

SAN BERNARDINO NATIONAL FOREST

RESTROOM

the mountains to Big Bear, remember the area's first tourists, who rode two days on burros up to the Bear Valley Hotel.

On the way home, drive the Rim of the World Highway (CA 38) to Redlands. Built in 1915, this road provided the first automobile access to Big Bear (no more burros!). The scenery is sensational.

GPS COORDINATES

UTM Zone (WGS84) 11S

Easting 502231

Northing 379411

Latitude N 34° 17' 17"

Longtitude W 116° 58' 33"

GETTING THERE

From L.A., go east on I-10, almost to San Bernardino. Then take CA 30 north to CA 330. About 35 miles later, you will arrive at the Big Bear Lake dam. Go left on CA 38 for 4 miles to Fawnskin. Turn left on Rim of the World Road. It becomes FS 3N14. Follow this dirt road a couple of miles to Hanna Flat Campground on the left.

47
HEART BAR CAMPGROUND

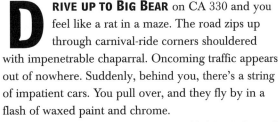

> *This is real mountain camping right near Los Angeles. Reserve for big holidays.*

DRIVE UP TO BIG BEAR on CA 330 and you feel like a rat in a maze. The road zips up through carnival-ride corners shouldered with impenetrable chaparral. Oncoming traffic appears out of nowhere. Suddenly, behind you, there's a string of impatient cars. You pull over, and they fly by in a flash of waxed paint and chrome.

You'll find a different scene on old CA 38, Rim of the World Scenic Highway. Drive out of Big Bear into a sea of granite and lodgepole pine and feast your eyes on "Greyback" himself, San Gorgonio Mountain at 11,502 feet (named for a very, very obscure Christian martyr). Come up from the bottom, from Redlands down in the desert, and suddenly you are in subalpine (boreal) forests of lodgepole pine twisted by the storms. The chaparral is high-altitude chaparral. There's manzanita, bush chinquapin, and snowbrush, plus all the alpine wildflowers. It's incredible! One moment you're driving through the mess of the city of San Bernardino, and the next you're in the splendor of the San Gorgonio Wilderness.

Heart Bar Campground is right in the belly of the beast. Why Heart Bar? It's a beautiful name. Here, in an area settled by pioneer Mormons, cattle herds were summered up in the meadows by the headwaters of the Santa Ana River. One of the local brands was the Heart Bar, a heart with a bar beneath it.

I love this campground. It's big and shaded, but it feels wide open. The meadow is green and bright in the sunlight. The pitches are clean and softened by pine needles. The sites are nicely spaced. And, the campground is not nearly as heavily used as nearby South Fork Campground, bunched along Lost Creek, or Barton Flats down below.

There is great hiking from the campground, stream fishing down by the South Fork Campground,

RATINGS

Beauty: ✩ ✩ ✩ ✩
Privacy: ✩ ✩ ✩ ✩
Spaciousness: ✩ ✩ ✩ ✩
Quiet: ✩ ✩ ✩ ✩ ✩
Security: ✩ ✩ ✩ ✩
Cleanliness: ✩ ✩ ✩ ✩ ✩

and lake fishing a short shot up at Big Bear Lake. At Big Bear, you can buy anything a body could need from big chain stores and little antique joints. Or, the other way, in Angelus Oaks, there's a general store as well as the Oaks Restaurant. You can also go farther and then left along Mill Creek to Forest Falls, where there is another general store.

For an easily accessed hike, head south a few hundred yards from Heart Bar Campground and connect with a trail that goes east to the headwaters of the Santa Ana River or west along its banks to South Fork Campground. Up here, the Santa Ana is a beautiful little stream flowing through meadows and forests of black oak, fir, and Jeffrey and ponderosa pine. Formed from natural springs and snowmelt, the Santa Ana River looks incredibly beautiful up here, yet hideously ugly down in Orange County in its concrete channel.

Or, hike up Wildhorse Creek. Walk out to the main road and go left. About 300 yards along you'll see a signed turnoff to the Wildhorse Trail on the right. Follow the dirt road up to a parking lot. The trail leaves from here. At first, it is an old road up through pines and juniper. Then it winds up a series of chaparral-covered ridges before going down into Wildhorse Creek Canyon. Walk about a mile and find Wildhorse Creek Trail Camp. Right now, you are about 3.5 miles out.

An ambitious hiker could continue and climb Sugar Loaf Mountain. Sugar Loaf has an elevation of about 9,952 feet and is a big lump on the divide between Big Bear country and the Santa Ana River Canyon. The best way is to hike up the saddle east of Sugar Loaf, then follow the trail along the ridgetop to the summit. I kept hearing about a famous, rare black butterfly and looked in vain for it when I was last there.

Another fun hike from Heart Bar Campground is to Aspen Grove. Go in the fall when the leaves are golden yellow. Head out of the campground to FS 1N02 (the road you drove in on). Turn right and walk about a mile to a fork in the road. Go right again and walk to a small parking lot near the signed trailhead for Aspen Grove Trail. Follow the old dirt road southeast to Fish Creek. Cross the creek and enjoy the

KEY INFORMATION

ADDRESS: Heart Bar Campground San Bernardino National Forest Mill Creek Ranger District 34701 Mill Creek Road Mentone, CA 92359

OPERATED BY: U.S. Forest Service

INFORMATION: (909) 794-1123; www.fs.fed.us/r5/ sanbernardino

OPEN: May 15–October 1

SITES: 95

EACH SITE HAS: Picnic table, fireplace

ASSIGNMENT: Some sites offer reservations; others are first come, first served.

REGISTRATION: At entrance (or with host); reserve by phone, (877) 444-6777, or online, www.reserveusa .com.

FACILITIES: Water, vault toilets

PARKING: At site

FEE: $10–$20; no fee for hiking, but auto touring costs $5 per day or $30 annually

ELEVATION: 7,000 feet

RESTRICTIONS: *Pets:* On leash only *Fires:* In fireplaces *Alcohol:* No restrictions *Vehicles:* RVs up to 50 feet long *Other:* Get a wilderness permit from Mill Creek Ranger Station.

MAP

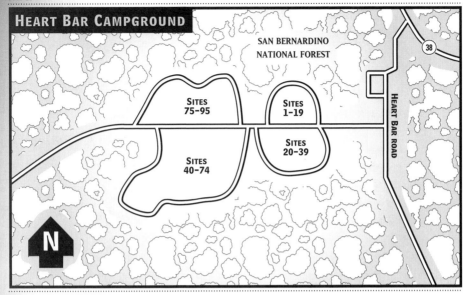

HEART BAR CAMPGROUND

SAN BERNARDINO
NATIONAL FOREST

38

SITES
75-95

SITES
1-19

SITES
20-39

SITES
40-74

HEART BAR ROAD

N

GETTING THERE

From L.A., go east on I-10 to Redlands past San Bernardino. Then take CA 38 east 33 miles to FS 1N02 and go right. The campground entrance is immediately on your right.

aspens—or what's left of them. Apparently, the California golden beaver enjoys them, too. A fellow hiker said that this particular beaver is not a San Bernardino native but was introduced by Forest Service wildlife experts who had not counted on the beaver's sudden passion for eating aspen.

Check out the dispersed camping in the area for future trips. Stop at the Mill Creek Ranger Station on CA 38 near the burg of Mentone. You'll need a wilderness permit for ambitious hiking anyway. Ask the ranger to show you where dispersed camping is allowed and where the yellow-post sites are. There is spectacular tent camping in the San Gorgonio area, and much of it is outside the organized campgrounds.

GPS COORDINATES

UTM Zone (WGS84) 11S

Easting 0519755

Northing 3780057

Latitude N 34° 9' 41"

Longtitude W 116° 47' 8"

48 LAGUNA CAMPGROUND

LAGUNA **C**AMPGROUND **OFFERS** some of the best camping in Southern California and the cheekiest ground squirrels and jays in the West. Hardly had my wife and I arrived at an incredible campsite on the edge of a yellow-flowered meadow stretching away to islands of pine against a cerulean blue sky, when a larcenous Stellar's jay swooped down on the picnic table and tried to take off with a particularly shiny spoon. Next, the California ground squirrels moved in for a package of corn chips on top of the cooler. I stomped my feet and threw gravel. They scurried a few feet away, rolled defiantly in the dust, and rose to attack the corn chips again. Then, I heard a shrill shriek, and the varmits scattered at the sight of a red-tailed hawk circling above.

Maintained by the Laguna Mountain Volunteer Association, Laguna Campground is clean and well run. There's a feeling of serenity and order. The little community of Laguna, with its stores, churches, fire department, restaurants, and rental cabins, reflects the pride of its residents. This is a very special place.

The campground is set in a meadow in a stand of Jeffrey pines, almost indistinguishable from ponderosa pines save the vanilla scent of their bark. Put your nose right up to the tree and take a whiff. Also, the bark on the Jeffrey tends toward narrow ridges, while ponderosa bark grows in large, flat plates. Roll the cones from a Jeffrey between your hands, and the spines won't prick—they are turned under. Ponderosa spines stick out.

Native Americans used the roots of Jeffrey pines to make baskets. They waited until the trees flowered and the roots were sufficiently tough. Then, they dug up the roots, cleaned, and slow-cooked them. Afterward, the roots were split and scraped until soft and pliable enough to weave.

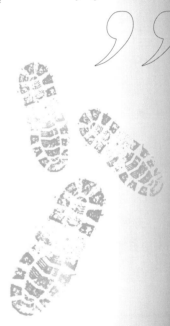

Laguna Campground is clean, well run, and near the proud community of Laguna.

RATINGS

Beauty: ✿ ✿ ✿ ✿ ✿
Privacy: ✿ ✿ ✿ ✿
Spaciousness: ✿ ✿ ✿ ✿
Quiet: ✿ ✿ ✿ ✿ ✿
Security: ✿ ✿ ✿ ✿ ✿
Cleanliness: ✿ ✿ ✿ ✿ ✿

KEY INFORMATION

ADDRESS:	Laguna Campground Cleveland National Forest Descanso Ranger District 3348 Alpine Boulevard Alpine, CA 91901
OPERATED BY:	U.S. Forest Service
INFORMATION:	Ranger Office: (619) 445-6235 or (619) 473-8824 (Monday–Friday, 8 a.m.–4:30 p.m.); visitor center: (619) 473-8547 (Friday–Sunday, May–September); www.fs.fed.us/r5/cleveland/recreation/camping/laguna.shtml
OPEN:	Year-round
SITES:	104 total; 30 tent-only
EACH SITE HAS:	Picnic table, fireplace
ASSIGNMENT:	Some sites offer reservations; others are walk-in.
REGISTRATION:	At entrance; reserve by phone, (877) 444-6777, or online, www.recreation.gov.
FACILITIES:	Water, vault toilets, showers
PARKING:	Near site
FEE:	$17
ELEVATION:	5,800 feet
RESTRICTIONS:	*Pets:* On leash only; must stay in tent or vehicle overnight *Fires:* In fireplace *Alcohol:* No restrictions *Vehicles:* RVs (maximum 25 feet), trailers

I met a German naturalist camping a few sites over who gave me the rundown on the squirrels. They are supposed to eat seeds, herbaceous vegetation, and acorns, but prefer to hang around campgrounds and eat corn chips. They hibernate in the winter; when spring comes, they have some catch-up eating to do. According to the naturalist, the shrill squeak I heard when the hawk cruised overhead was from the oldest squirrel in the colony. Apparently, the squirrel who sounds the alarm has the greatest chance of being picked off by the hawk. So, the oldest squirrel protects his own offspring, and the band, by sounding the alarm and offering himself as the victim if need be. Pretty brave stuff for the little guy.

In the meadow by the campground is Little Laguna Lake. Little more than a wallow, it is still home to many waterfowl and loudly croaking frogs. A kopje (stand of rocks in a meadow) nearby is a convenient place to sit and watch the wildlife through binoculars. The meadow was carpeted with tiny sunflowers, tidy tips, Achilles's fern, and the edible miner's lettuce when I visited in June.

We picked up a trail to Big Laguna Lake to the south of the campground. The trail meanders for about a mile across meadows and along the edge of the pined hummocks that beg for picnickers. Big Laguna Lake, which is only a lake indeed in the spring and summer of wet years, was big and beautiful on our visit. From the lake, the mostly flat trail turns north and connects with Noble Canyon Trail and Pine Creek Road.

If you want a desert view, trade the pines of Laguna for the oaks of Burnt Rancheria Campground a few miles south, also run by the Laguna Mountain Volunteer Society.

Laguna Campground is open all year (Burnt Rancheria is open May to October), but I think spring is the best time to visit. In winter, there's snow and snow sports, but half of San Diego flocks here on wintry weekends. Summers get a bit hot and dusty. Both campgrounds are popular, so plan on getting here Friday by noon if you don't have a reservation.

While visiting, run down to Tecate, Mexico (a half-hour to the south). Or, take I-8 to Anza-Borrego

MAP

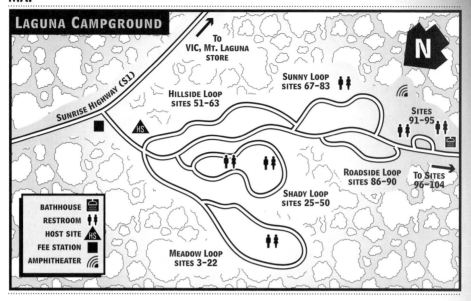

LAGUNA CAMPGROUND

To VIC, MT. LAGUNA STORE

SUNNY LOOP SITES 67-83

SUNRISE HIGHWAY (S1)

HILLSIDE LOOP SITES 51-63

SITES 91-95

N

ROADSIDE LOOP SITES 86-90

To SITES 96-104

SHADY LOOP SITES 25-50

MEADOW LOOP SITES 3-22

BATHHOUSE
RESTROOM
HOST SITE HS
FEE STATION
AMPHITHEATER

Desert State Park or the Sunrise Highway north to Julian to fish in Lake Cuyamaca. There is a lot to do around here. Go horseback riding or mountain biking. Stargaze from the night-sky observatories at the south end of the recreation area. This is a wonderful part of Southern California.

GETTING THERE

From San Diego, drive 50 miles east on I-8 to the Laguna Junction exit. Drive 11 miles farther north on Sunrise Highway to Mount Laguna, then 2.5 miles north to the signed entrance on the left marked "Laguna/ El Prado." Laguna is the campground you want.

GPS COORDINATES

UTM Zone (WGS84) 11S
Easting 551523
Northing 3639004
Latitude N 32 ° 53' 17"
Longtitude W 116° 26' 57"

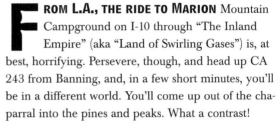

> *Marion Mountain, nestled in the clouds, is a great break from nearby Los Angeles.*

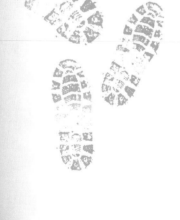

FROM L.A., THE RIDE TO MARION Mountain Campground on I-10 through "The Inland Empire" (aka "Land of Swirling Gases") is, at best, horrifying. Persevere, though, and head up CA 243 from Banning, and, in a few short minutes, you'll be in a different world. You'll come up out of the chaparral into the pines and peaks. What a contrast!

Marion Mountain Campground is as sunny and airy as nearby Dark Canyon Campground is dark and safe, down under sheltering trees. Between the two, you'll see the entire spectrum of good San Jacinto tent camping.

The access road to Marion Mountain Campground from CA 243 is narrow and winding. This cuts down on the trailers and RVs. The site parking spaces are short—about 15 feet tops. The picnic tables and fireplaces are down in the trees away from the parking area. All this discourages RVers and gives an edge to tent campers.

The water from a spring above the campground is good. Let the tap run for a moment to clear any sediment if the campground has been lightly used. All the facilities are well maintained. The pit-toilet bathrooms are surprisingly clean, and tiled on the floors and walls. I wanted to stay for a week. When you first arrive at Marion Mountain Campground, it's difficult to locate the sites. This is because most of them are isolated from each other among the pines. The pitches, on pine needles, are nice and spongy. Through the pine boughs, you'll see the steep slopes of the mountains across the canyon, all covered with pines, oaks, and rocky tors.

I brought along a portable radio/cassette player with a few classical music tapes. What a wonderful experience! Camping in the mountains goes with classical music. A music professor once told me that music

RATINGS

Beauty: ✪ ✪ ✪
Privacy: ✪ ✪ ✪ ✪ ✪
Spaciousness: ✪ ✪ ✪ ✪ ✪
Quiet: ✪ ✪ ✪ ✪ ✪
Security: ✪ ✪ ✪ ✪ ✪
Cleanliness: ✪ ✪ ✪ ✪ ✪

began when primitive man, imbued with the "like produces like" principle, endeavored to wake the sleeping
earth from its winter nap by beating it with a stick in
the spring. From this came the percussion drums and
then the more sophisticated woodwinds that imitated
the birds.

To hike from the campground, go to Site 12.
Across from that site's picnic table, there is a dirt road
that heads up the slope. Follow it for 20 yards and
notice the trail arrows pointing right and left. The right
arrows lead you down the hill to the trailhead. The left
ones indicate the Marion Mountain Trail, which goes
up into the State Park and joins the Pacific Crest Trail
near Deer Spring. It climbs the heavily forested northwest flank of Marion Mountain and is the shortest way
to climb San Jacinto Peak.

Take plenty of water and be aware of thunderstorms. When there is lightning, avoid open areas like
meadows, ridges, and mountaintops. Stay away from
isolated trees and take cover under dense, small trees
in lower areas, in a boulder field, or in a cave. Failing
all this, lie flat on the ground. And, in all cases, remove
metal-frame backpacks and metal tent poles. Really,
lightning is no joke. I suffered a near miss in the
Mojave Desert a few summers ago. It burned my
calves and scared me half to death.

In early September, when I last visited Marion
Mountain, there were thunderstorm clouds over the
mountains. The dry air carried a hint of rain. As we
were hiking up the slopes around the campground,
there was a roll of thunder, and a splatter of rain hit
the dusty rocks. What drama! The campground host
told me they'd had a hard storm hit in the middle of
August. It rained like hell for a couple of hours, and
then the sun came out. This is typical of the Southern
Sierras in late August and September, and something
to watch for.

A good place for a sundowner is up the dirt road
across from Site 12. Go past the arrows for the Marion
Mountain Trail. About 20 yards up, climb the ridge to
the right, and there are some nice big boulders to sit
on and watch the sun set. Back on the dirt road, walk
to the end of it. There's a short trail that switchbacks

KEY INFORMATION

ADDRESS:	Marion Mountain Campground San Bernardino National Forest
OPERATED BY:	U.S. Forest Service
INFORMATION:	(909) 382-2921; www.fs.fed.us/r5/ sanbernardino/ recreation/camping/ index.shtml
OPEN:	May–mid-October
SITES:	24
EACH SITE HAS:	Picnic table, fire pit
ASSIGNMENT:	Some sites offer reservations; others are first come, first served.
REGISTRATION:	At entrance; reserve by phone, (877) 444-6777, or online, www.recreation.gov.
FACILITIES:	Water, pit toilets
PARKING:	Near site
FEE:	$10; $5 for extra vehicle
ELEVATION:	6,400 feet
RESTRICTIONS:	*Pets:* On leash only *Fires:* In fire pit *Alcohol:* No restrictions *Vehicles:* No RVs longer than 15 feet *Other:* No dogs allowed within Mount San Jacinto State Park wilder- ness; permits are required to enter wilderness.

MAP

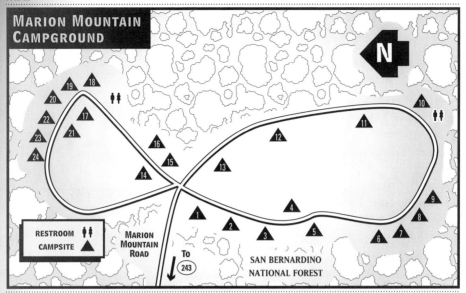

MARION MOUNTAIN CAMPGROUND

N

RESTROOM
CAMPSITE

MARION MOUNTAIN ROAD

To 243

SAN BERNARDINO NATIONAL FOREST

GETTING THERE

From L.A., drive east to Banning. Go south on CA 243 for 22 miles. Turn left at FS 4S02 and drive 1.7 miles to the campground.

up the slope to some cabins, where there is an incredible view of the southwest side of the range.

Head south to Pine Cove to find gas and ice. For a town with everything, go a few miles farther to Idyllwild, a lovely little mountain town. Idyllwild even has a shopping center with a supermarket and a hardware store. They have butchers, restaurants, artists, writers, and, of course, the San Jacinto Ranger Station—to the left as you enter town. If Marion Mountain and the other campgrounds nearby are full, or if you want to disperse-camp or yellow-post-camp, that's where you need to go. The rangers will fix you up with a fire permit and show you where to go.

GPS COORDINATES

UTM Zone (WGS84) 11S
Easting 524850
Northing 3739121
Latitude N 33° 47' 31"
Longtitude W 116° 43' 54"

50
WILLIAM HEISE COUNTY PARK CAMPGROUND

AMONG THE MANY REASONS to tent-camp in William Heise County Park are the incredible drives in from L.A. via Warner Springs or from San Diego via Ramona or Cuyamaca Rancho State Park. All three show Southern California at its most charming and very best—the rolling, forested hills, the green meadows, the tiny western towns. This was the real gold the forty-niners found when they arrived in California—this beautiful land. On all three drives, near Julian, you climb 2 miles south on Pine Hills Road, then left on Frisius Drive. Those final 2 miles carry you through farmland that echoes bucolic Vermont or New Hampshire. The resemblance is eerie. You can only imagine the argonauts; after walking 3,000 miles across the continent they must have looked around Frisius Drive and thought, "My God! I'm home."

Made up of 900 acres of oak, pine, and cedar, William Heise County Park is upper chaparral; this area is also known as cold chaparral because most of the precipitation comes from snow and fog drip. As you hike around and in the park, watch the slope orientation to see the effect.

On south-facing slopes there are evergreen shrubs with thick oval leaves like the manzanita. Note how the manzanita leaves are mealy and waxy and are often oriented vertically to reduce the amount of light that directly strikes the leaf surface.

Manzanita endure droughts, resist fire, and withstand cold. On north-facing slopes look for California live oak; Jeffrey, Coulter, sugar, and ponderosa pines; white fir; and incense cedar.

Like Cuyamaca Rancho State Park, William Heise is a birder's paradise. Look for various hawks, eagles, owls, woodpeckers, vireos, warblers, sparrows, and the like. Also, look for the full complement of Southern California reptiles and various rodents eating the

> *Visit California high country and feel like you're in Vermont at the same time.*

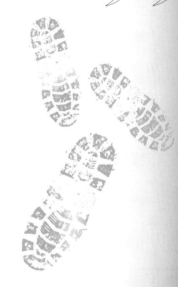

RATINGS

Beauty: ✩ ✩ ✩ ✩
Privacy: ✩ ✩
Spaciousness: ✩ ✩ ✩
Quiet: ✩ ✩ ✩
Security: ✩ ✩ ✩
Cleanliness: ✩ ✩ ✩

plethora of acorns. Acorns were a Cahuilla Native American staple, made into meal and then bread.

Once, camping at William Heise, we experimented with acorn bread. First, we ground the acorns into a coarse meal, then, following local Cahuilla recipe, we filled a colander with fine sand, patted the coarsely ground acorn meal down into a bowl-like depression in the sand, and poured water slowly over the meal to leach out the bitterness. Then we pounded the meal down finer in a mortar until it resembled a fine powder. Finally, the meal was sifted, mixed with water, and baked on a hot rock: not bad, but a little bitter.

Encouraged, my camping companion resolved to fatten up a pig on the acorns in his yard at home. He found a candidate piglet and penned it up under his oak trees. For weeks, it ate acorns heartily. Then, a carelessly guarded plate of chicken enchiladas and refried beans was left out. The pig got it, and that was it; his palate was ruined. No more acorns. He rejected Native American cuisine, and finally became Thanksgiving dinner himself.

Heise is a friendly place to camp. Almost half of the sites are for tents only, which separates you from the RVs that feel like city blocks on wheels when you're lying there in a little tent. The park is roomy, and the restrooms are very clean. Once, we rented one of the two rental cabins at Heise. It had six wooden bunks and a maximum capacity of eight ($35 per night plus reservation fee). Bring your own bedding and a padlock for the door. Cooking is done outside on a barbecue. It was as jolly as a good school trip. For reservations, call (858) 565-3600.

Heise is a fine base camp from which to explore Julian, Wynola, and Santa Ysabel. Do an apple pie comparison test. Stop for a drink or breakfast at the much-fabled Pine Hills Lodge by the junction of Pine Hills Road and Frisius Drive. Visit the Santa Ysabel Mission 2 miles north of Santa Ysabel on CA 79. See the museum in Julian. Take the Eagle Mine tour. Ask the ranger or campground host at Heise about trips to Boulder Creek and Boulder Creek Falls. Don't miss a killer hike (11 miles round-trip) down Kelly Ditch Trail to Cuyamaca Rancho State Park.

MAP

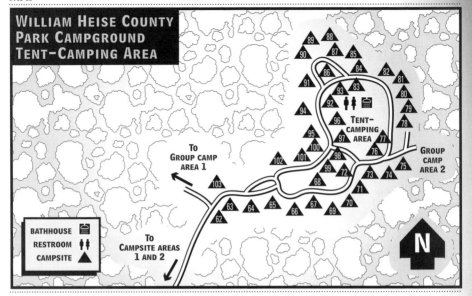

WILLIAM HEISE COUNTY PARK CAMPGROUND TENT-CAMPING AREA

To GROUP CAMP AREA 1

TENT-CAMPING AREA

GROUP CAMP AREA 2

BATHHOUSE
RESTROOM
CAMPSITE

To CAMPSITE AREAS 1 AND 2

N

GETTING THERE

From L.A., take I-10 east to I-15. Go south to Temecula. Take CA 79 southeast to Santa Ysabel. Go left toward Julian 5.8 miles to Pine Hills Road. Go right and drive 2 miles to Frisius Drive and make a left. Go 2 miles, and you are at the park.

MAP

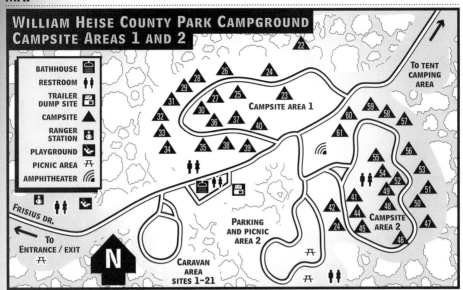

GPS COORDINATES

UTM Zone (WGS84) 11S

Easting 538410

Northing 3655816

Latitude N 33° 02' 25"

Longtitude W 116° 35' 19"

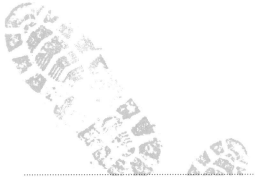

APPENDIXES

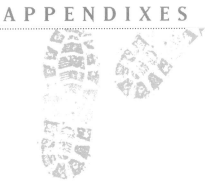

APPENDIX A
CAMPING-EQUIPMENT CHECKLIST

Except for the large and bulky items on this list, I keep a plastic storage container full of the essentials of car camping so that they're ready to go when I am. I make a last-minute check of the inventory, resupply anything that's low or missing, and away I go.

COOKING UTENSILS
Bottle opener
Bottles of salt, pepper, spices, sugar, cooking oil, and maple syrup in waterproof, spill-proof containers
Can opener
Corkscrew
Cups, plastic or tin
Dish soap (biodegradable), sponge, towel
Flatware
Food of your choice
Frying pan
Fuel for stove
Matches in waterproof container
Plates
Pocketknife
Pot with lid
Spatula
Stove
Tin foil
Wooden spoon

FIRST-AID KIT
Antibiotic cream
Aspirin or ibuprofen
Band-Aids®
Diphenhydramine (Benadryl®)
Gauze pads
Insect repellent
Moleskin®
Snakebite kit (if you're heading for desert conditions)
Sunscreen/lip balm
Tape, waterproof adhesive
Tweezers

SLEEPING GEAR
Pillow
Sleeping bag
Sleeping pad, inflatable or insulated
Tent with ground tarp and rainfly

MISCELLANEOUS
Bath soap (biodegradable), washcloth, towel
Camp chair
Candles
Cellular phone
Cooler
Deck of cards
Fire starter
Flashlight or headlamp with fresh batteries
Foul-weather clothing (useful year-round in the Northwest)
Lantern
Paper towels
Plastic zip-top bags
Sunglasses
Toilet paper
Water bottle
Wool blanket

OPTIONAL
Barbecue grill
Binoculars
Field guides on bird, plant, and wildlife identification
Fishing rod and tackle
GPS
Hatchet
Maps (road, topographic, trails, etc.)

APPENDIX B
SUGGESTED READING
AND REFERENCE

The Anza-Borrego Desert Region. Lindsay, Lowell and Diana. Wilderness Press, 1998.

Best Short Hikes in California's Northern Sierra. Whitehill, Karen and Terry. The Mountaineers, 1990.

Best Short Hikes in California's Southern Sierra. Whitehill, Karen and Terry. The Mountaineers, 1991.

California Camping. Stienstra, Tom. Foghorn Press, 2003.

California's Desert Trails. Chase, J. Smeaton. Tioga Publishing Co., 1987.

California's Eastern Sierra. Irwin, Sue. Cachuma Press, 1992.

Day Hiker's Guide to Southern California. McKinney, John. Olympus Press, 1998.

Day Hiking Kings Canyon. Sorensen, Steve. Fuyu Press, 1992.

Day Hiking Sequoia. Sorensen, Steve. Fuyu Press, 1996.

Exploring the Southern Sierra: East Side. Jenkins, J. C. and Ruby Johnson. Jenkins and Jenkins, 1991.

Exploring the Southern Sierra: West Side. Jenkins, J. C. and Ruby Johnson. Jenkins and Jenkins, 1995.

Gem Trails of Southern California. Mitchell, James R. Gem Guides Book Co., 2003.

Gold! Gold! Petralia, Joseph F. Sierra Outdoor Products Co., 1996.

A Natural History of California. Schoenherr, Allan A. University of California Press, 1995.

Roadside Plants of Southern California. Belzer, Thomas J. Mountain Press, 2003.

San Bernardino Mountain Trails. Robinson, John W. Wilderness Press, 2003.

A Treasury of the Sierra Nevada. Reid, Robert Leonard. Wilderness Press, 1983.

Walking California's State Parks. McKinney, John. Olympus Press, 2000.

APPENDIX C
SOURCES OF INFORMATION

B.L.M., CALIFORNIA STATE OFFICE
2800 Cottage Way, Suite W1834
Sacramento, CA 95825-1886
(916) 978-4400
www.ca.blm.gov

CALIFORNIA STATE PARKS
P.O. Box 942896
Sacramento, CA 94296
(916) 653-6995
www.parks.ca.gov

DEATH VALLEY NATIONAL PARK
P.O. Box 579
Death Valley, CA 92328
(760) 786-3200
www.nps.gov/deva

INYO NATIONAL FOREST
351 Pacu Lane, Suite 200
Bishop, CA 93514
(760) 873-2400
www.fs.fed.us/r5/inyo

JOSHUA TREE NATIONAL PARK
74485 National Park Drive
Twentynine Palms, CA 92277-3597
(760) 367-5500
www.nps.gov/jotr

LOS PADRES NATIONAL FOREST
6755 Hollister Avenue, Suite 150
Goleta, CA 93117
(805) 968-6640
www.fs.fed.us/r5/lospadres

MOJAVE NATIONAL PRESERVE
222 East. Main Street, Suite 202
Barstow, CA 92311
(760) 255-8800
www.nps.gov/moja

NATIONAL PARK SERVICE, PACIFIC WEST REGION
1111 Jackson Street, Suite 700
Oakland, CA 94607
(510) 817-1300
www.nps.gov

PINNACLES CAMPGROUND, INC.
2400 Highway 146
Paicines, CA 95043
(831) 389-4462
www.pinncamp.com

PINNACLES NATIONAL MONUMENT
5000 Highway 146
Paicines, CA 95043
(831) 389-4485
www.nps.gov/pinn

SAN BERNARDINO NATIONAL FOREST
S. 1824 Commercenter Circle
San Bernardino, CA 92408-3430
(909) 382-2600
www.fs.fed.us/r5/sanbernardino

SEQUOIA AND KINGS CANYON NATIONAL PARK
47050 Generals Highway
Three Rivers, CA 93271-9651
(559) 565-3341
www.nps.gov/seki

SEQUOIA NATIONAL FOREST
900 West Grand Avenue
Porterville, CA 93257
(559) 784-1500
www.fs.fed.us/r5/sequoia

APPENDIX C
SOURCES OF INFORMATION

SIERRA NATIONAL FOREST
1600 Tollhouse Road
Clovis, CA 93611-0532
(559) 297-0706
www.fs.fed.us/r5/sierra

YOSEMITE NATIONAL PARK
P.O. Box 577
Yosemite National Park, CA 95389
(209) 372-0200
www.nps.gov/yose

U.S. FOREST SERVICE,
PACIFIC SOUTHWEST REGION
1323 Club Drive
Vallejo, CA 94592
(707) 562.8737
www.fs.fed.us/r5

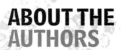

BILL MAI

Working for the Denver Museum of Natural History, Bill's mother was an avid camper, and she developed in her son a love for the outdoors. Inspired by the Native American "digs" that his mother worked on and their many camping jaunts to Maine, the Adirondacks, and numerous locations in the West, Bill continued to foster his enthusiasm for camping.

Bill lived in Santa Monica, California, where he wrote screenplays and wonderful books about his love of camping, including *The Best in Tent Camping: Northern California,* the series counterpart to this book. He currently resides in Winston-Salem, North Carolina.

CHARLES PATTERSON

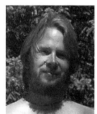A Southern California native, Charles daydreams about his next outdoor adventure every time he finds himself indoors, bound by some professional or otherwise mundane obligation. Naturally, he relishes the opportunity to explore further, pushing himself to greater lengths than most would tolerate. Writing *Mountain Bike! Los Angeles County: A Wide-Grin Ride Guide* forced Charles to spend many hours in the sticks, often alone, occasional pondering the size of local mountain-lion populations. It was a true adventure, and getting to write about it afterward and share his love for the outdoors was a blessing. Revising *The Best in Tent Camping: Southern California* is a natural progression, because Charles's banged-up body certainly can't tolerate two-wheeled pursuits forever, and tent camping is an activity he'll still be able to enjoy after his first walker, cane, or wheelchair purchase.

INDEX

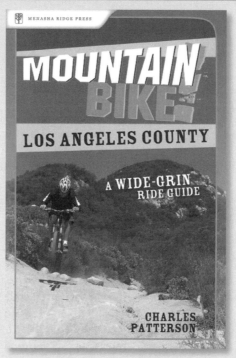

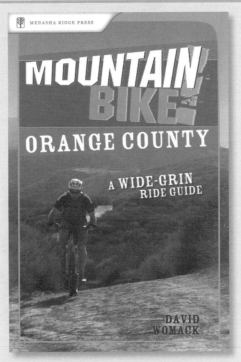

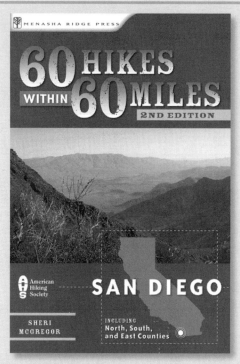